Coping with Vision Loss

DISCARD

Ordering

Trade bookstores in the U.S. and Canada, please contact:

Publishers Group West
1700 Fourth Street, Berkeley CA 94710
Phone: (800) 788-3123   Fax: (510) 528-3444

Hunter House books are available at bulk discounts for textbook course adoptions; to qualifying community, health care, and government organizations; and for special promotions and fund-raising. For details please contact:

Special Sales Department
Hunter House Inc., PO Box 2914, Alameda CA 94501-0914
Phone: (510) 865-5282   Fax: (510) 865-4295
E-mail: ordering@hunterhouse.com

Individuals can order our books from most bookstores or by calling toll-free:
(800) 266-5592

Coping with Vision Loss

Maximizing What You Can See and Do

Bill G. Chapman

Doctor of Rehabilitation Psychology and
Rehabilitation Administration

Illustrated by George H. Pollock

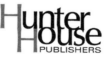

Hunter House Inc., Publishers
PO Box 2914
Alameda CA 94501-0914

Library of Congress Cataloging-in-Publication Data

Chapman, Bill G.
Coping with vision loss : maximizing what you can see and do /
Bill G. Chapman
    p. cm.
Includes bibliographical references and index.
ISBN 0-89793-316-8 (pb.) — ISBN 0-89793-317-6 (cl.)
    1. Vision disorders—Popular works. 2. Low vision—Popular works. 3. Large type books. I. Title.
RE51 .C48 2001
617.7—dc21   00-054688

Project Credits

Cover Design: Jinni Fontana
Book Production: Hunter House
Developmental and Copy Editor: Kelley Blewster
Proofreader: Lee Rappold
Indexer: Kathy Talley-Jones
Graphics Assistance: Ariel Parker, Jil Weil
Acquisitions Editor: Jeanne Brondino
Associate Editor: Alexandra Mummery
Editorial and Production Assistant: Melissa Millar
Publicity Manager: Sarah Frederick
Marketing Assistant: Earlita Chenault
Customer Service Manager: Christina Sverdrup
Order Fulfillment: Joel Irons
Administrator: Theresa Nelson
Computer Support: Peter Eichelberger
Publisher: Kiran S. Rana

Printed and Bound by Publishers Press, Salt Lake City, Utah

Manufactured in the United States of America

9 8 7 6 5 4 3 2 1   First Edition   01 02 03 04 05

A note about the design of the book

This book has been typeset to make it easier to read for people with vision impairment. It features larger than usual type sizes and vertical spacing, typefaces selected for easy readability, the use of **bold** and <u>underlined</u> instead of italic fonts, unjustified text so the word spacing does not vary too much, extra wide inside margins, and simple layouts. While it does not conform to the specifications for a large-type book, we feel this "in-between" design allows us to make the information available to a wider audience — including family members and medical professionals who would benefit from this information — while at the same time supporting our primary objective of making this information accessible to people with severe vision loss.

Disclaimer

The material in this book is intended to provide a review of resources and information related to vision loss. Every effort has been made to provide accurate and dependable information. However, professionals in the field may have differing opinions, and change is always taking place. Any of the treatments described herein should be followed under the guidance of a licensed health care practitioner.

The publisher, authors, editors, and professionals quoted in the book cannot be held responsible for any error, omission, professional disagreement, outdated material, or adverse outcomes that derive from the use of any of the treatments or information resources in this book. Always check all questions and treatments with a qualified health care professional.

Contents

A Matter of Perspective: How to Use This Book
The Scope of the Book

PART I: Vision and the Human Eye

"Legal Blindness" Defined
How Test Charts Mislead
Visual Impairment Defined
A Visual Disability Scale
Disability: Handicap or Challenge?
Testing Your Visual Acuity

The Eyeball's Shape
A. The Cornea
B. The Iris
C. The Lens
D. The Retina

PART III: Major Causes of Vision Loss

PART IV: Coping Techniques and Equipment

PART V: Specialized Knowledge and Skills

List of Illustrations

Acknowledgments

I am indebted to many people for help in writing this book. At the top of the list is my wife, Katherine, who proofread the manuscript repeatedly, correcting errors my vision failed to detect.

Special thanks go to Dr. Don Swick and Dr. Lin Moore, who are pioneers in the field of low-vision services. Both have prescribed aids that have kept me functional for the past twenty-nine years. Naturally, I turned to them for technical assistance when this book was first written. They graciously read the manuscript and made suggestions that were gratefully accepted.

Foreword

Dear Reader:

I have been a Doctor of Optometry for over fifty years. I grew up in a home with a partially blind sister. These two facts have combined to give me a special interest in working with low-vision patients.

You are holding in your hands a practical, down-to-earth blueprint for making life more complete and enjoyable. In it, I describe exact ways of dealing with the various frustrations of visual handicaps are described.

Some brilliant doctors like Dr. Chapman confine their skills to writing textbooks about current research for students and other doctors. This book, however, is based on his years of experience in dealing personally with his own loss of vision due to a form of macular degeneration called Stargardt's disease. Combining this frightening experience with years of study and a full measure of common sense, Dr. Chapman could visualize the advantages of taking his personal knowledge of the need for services to the persons who needed them. Dr. Chapman took to the road in a van equipped with various models of closed-circuit television sets, large-print books, magnifying devices, electronic vision enhancers, cooking aids, and other household tools designed to assist those with limited vision.

As he visited in doctors' offices and people's homes, discussing the needs of both visually impaired persons and their family members, he began to see a growing need for this book. You are so fortunate that he took years of research and experience to write this for you and your families. I finally have a guidebook to recommend to my patients that will truly help.

As with most worthwhile things, you must work for the results promoted in this book. Doing so may not be easy, but here is the blueprint. Read it, study it, follow it.

Lin Moore, O.D., Low-Vision Specialist

Introduction

<u>Coping with Vision Loss: Maximizing What You Can See and Do</u> is about vision rehabilitation, a process that teaches and equips a sufferer of partial vision loss to use his or her remaining vision to function as a sighted person. Vision rehabilitation differs from rehabilitation of the blind. Vision rehabilitation begins with a person who is visually impaired but still enjoys some useful vision, whereas rehabilitation of the blind seeks to train and equip a totally blind person to function without vision.

Often, a person suffering from visual impairment considers himself or herself the most horribly handicapped person on earth. Surely, he or she feels, no one is worse off. This attitude stems from the very personal nature of vision loss, and while it is understandable and in many ways justifiable, it enables such people to believe they are beyond hope of vision rehabilitation. Such a desperate perspective is unnecessary. Many sufferers of partial vision loss can be helped by the processes described in this book. For the purposes of this book, I define a candidate for vision rehabilitation as follows: If a person can see light, modern technology can help him or her to use that vision effectively. If a person can walk around an unfamiliar room avoiding almost all of the furniture, he or she is a prime candidate for vision rehabilitation.

I take great pleasure in conducting this tour of vision rehabilitation. I do so not from the standpoint of an ophthalmologist or optometrist, but rather as a member of that singular population known as the partially sighted. For thirty-four years I have faced the emotional trauma of vision loss and have experienced the frustration of losing skills I held dear. Like others, I came to think less of myself because I could no longer do the things I had formerly been able to. I had spent eight years training for the ministry. That path was gone, because I could no longer read. I spent four more years in postgraduate school, earning a doctorate in rehabilitation and psychology. Even that didn't prove viable. One hundred and fifty potential employers turned down my application for work. Halfway through the doctoral program I learned about vision rehabilitation. The discovery changed my life, gave me hope. What a beautiful message! Persons with only a little vision could still function sighted. I had been a minister of the Gospel; I became an evangelist of vision rehabilitation. What I learned from personal experience has been augmented by my purposeful study of the subject, knowledge gleaned from low-vision specialists like Dr. Don Swick and Dr. Lin Moore. With their help I learned how to help myself and others.

The journey of learning to cope with significant vision loss may lead readers into deep, dark valleys where it seems that terror, depression, and frustration crouch like tigers ready to spring. Fortunately, the path also leads to peaks where the air is clean and fresh and the sun shines brightly in a cloudless sky. On those peaks the reader will find a treasure: a way of minimizing the effects of the disease that has destroyed his or her vision. I wrote <u>Coping with Vision Loss</u> to be a roadmap out of the valleys and a guide for scaling the peaks.

A Matter of Perspective: How to Use This Book

Give two thirsty people half a glass of water. One joyfully announces, "My glass is half full!" The other mournfully mutters,

"My glass is half empty." This classic illustration of the difference between optimists and pessimists applies when it comes to vision rehabilitation. Consider the following.

Several years ago on a winter day, I was working with visually impaired seniors at a retirement center in south Texas. I showed a man in his seventies a pair of amber glasses that cost about four dollars. The glasses helped him, so he bought them.

He put them on and walked to his duplex three hundred yards away. By the time he reached his front door, he knew he had found the greatest low-vision aid in the world. He marveled at the detail they helped him to see. Then he began to worry. What if he broke this pair of marvelous glasses? What if he misplaced them? Where could he find another pair? He turned around and ran all the way back to the main building in the hope of catching me before I left. The man bought a backup pair and went home happy.

By contrast, other visually impaired seniors at the retirement home tried the same glasses. They took a brief look and then removed them, saying, "They don't help me very much," so they didn't buy them.

The difference in the two perspectives is a matter of mindset. Amber lenses help everyone, even the normally sighted. They increase contrast, making objects easier to see. This is a scientific fact. The first man rejoiced because the glasses helped him to see better. The others were looking for a miracle that would fully restore their lost vision. The amber lenses couldn't do that, so they rejected the improvement provided by the contrast-enhancing lenses.

The person who reads this book looking for a magic wand — a secret potion, a miracle cure that will suddenly and spontaneously restore complete vision — is wasting his time. This material can't help that person, because there is no such cure or easy way out.

Reading this book expecting to find a miracle on the next page sets the stage for failure. People with this mindset can't help themselves. Doctors can't help them, and even science can't.

On the other hand, help exists for those who are willing to learn how to use light properly. Add to this the knowledge of how contrast enhancement helps everyone. Take a giant step and use magnification correctly. Master eccentric viewing and scanning methods, and then combine all these techniques. Most persons with visual impairment can regain independence and privacy. All will be able to do more than they thought they could.

Except in the case of cataracts, vision lost to disease can rarely be regained. Even if a cure for the disease is found, the vision a person has already lost will not be restored, but by combining techniques discussed in <u>Coping with Vision Loss</u>, these persons can minimize their disability. If the reader embraces the skills and coping techniques discussed in this book, he or she can overcome or minimize the devastating impact of vision loss.

Permit me to offer some practical tips for using this book. As with any subject, vision rehabilitation has its own unique vocabulary. Every person with visual impairment should know certain terms that are commonly used. When one of these terms appears in this book, I define and explain it. Thereafter, it is assumed that the term is understood. For this reason, it may be most helpful to read straight through the book.

The book provides prices for various aids. The prices, in effect at the time of publication, may quickly become out-of-date; nevertheless, they will offer a general idea even if the book is read years after publication.

In some cases, I recommend specific aids by brand name and model number. If a product is recommended by name, it is because my experience is that it offers almost universal application and is as good as or better than other aids in that class. The primary purpose of this approach is not to discriminate against any given manufacturer, but to provide at least one specific aid the reader can locate.

There are five endnotes in the book. They are numbered consecutively and can be found on page 273.

The Scope of the Book

Coping with vision loss, or vision rehabilitation, involves several things:

1. Patients need to know certain things about their eyes and vision.

2. They need to know exactly what part of their vision they are losing.

3. They need to know the techniques used to overcome the effects of the disease. In some cases, special skills must be learned. Needed skills extend beyond learning to use specific aids. They may include learning to use the eyes differently from the way normally sighted individuals do.

4. Some people need specialized knowledge to cope with special needs. The two most common problems relate to getting an education and driving.

I address each of these concerns in this book.

A person can lose vision from many causes. Coping with Vision Loss concentrates on five of the leading ones: cataracts, diabetic retinopathy, glaucoma, macular degeneration, and retinitis pigmentosa. These five conditions cover a wide range of vision loss. Those uncertain about which disease is destroying their vision, or about the disease's precise effects, should obtain such information from their doctor. Ask the doctor if the condition is similar in its destructive effects to one of the major causes of vision loss discussed in this book. Such knowledge will help you to identify which information in the book is applicable to your situation.

Diabetic retinopathy and retinitis pigmentosa can destroy all of one's vision. Cataracts and glaucoma can do the same. Persons who have reached that point are candidates for blind rehabilitation, a topic outside the scope of this book.

Besides knowing **what** is destroying vision, persons should know **how** it happens. For the most part, this book summarizes how the five diseases mentioned above destroy vision, but it does not provide a detailed discussion. Again, talk to a trusted doctor about these matters if you want more details.

One **can** cope with vision loss! Even though, in most cases, neither medicine nor surgery can restore sight, a sufferer of partial vision loss **can** improve his or her situation. True, the better one's vision, the better one can function, but even a person with severe loss can improve functional ability when he or she knows how. Approached with an open mind and with a willingness to see the glass half full, Coping with Vision Loss tells you how.

Part I

Vision and the Human Eye

CHAPTER 1

Visual Acuity

Visual acuity notation — the pair of numerals that tell you how well (or otherwise) you can see — will be used in this book, so readers need to know exactly what the numbers mean. With this knowledge, a person with a degenerative disease can keep track of his or her vision loss.

A legally blind person has a visual acuity of 20/200 or worse, which would be indicated by a second number larger than 200, for example, 20/350. Just what do these numbers mean?

Notice that the numbers are written as a fraction. They consist of a numerator and a denominator. The numerator, or first number, is usually 20. This refers to 20 feet — the distance we sit from the test chart when the doctor tests our vision. The standard is to use 20 feet, but when working with persons who have subnormal vision, doctors sometimes use 10 feet, 5 feet, or even 1 foot. The distance in feet between the patient and the test chart becomes the numerator of his or her visual acuity.

The denominator, or second number, refers to the size of the letters on the test chart. They are a very specific size. If a letter is the 200-size, it means someone with normal vision (20/20) can read that size letter from 200 feet away. A person with normal vision can read 60-size and 120-size letters from a distance of 60 and 120 feet respectively.

The big "E" at the top of the test chart is usually a 200-size letter. A visual acuity of 20/200 means that while one person must

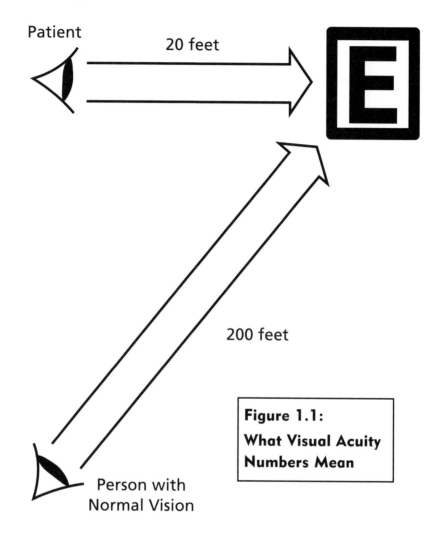

Patient

20 feet

200 feet

Figure 1.1:
What Visual Acuity
Numbers Mean

Person with
Normal Vision

sit 20 feet from the chart to read the big "E," someone who has normal vision can sit 200 feet from the chart and read the same-size letter. Neither of them would be able to read a smaller-size letter from these distances: keep this in mind while reading the book.

The following is key to understanding visual acuity. A person standing 20 feet from the chart who reads the 200-size letter will be able to read a 100-size letter when he moves to 10 feet from the chart. So, 20/200, 10/100, 5/50, and 2/20 all indicate the same visual acuity. The ratio between the numerator and denominator is 1/10 in all these cases. This concept is discussed more fully in Chapter 13.

The reader should understand that this material is theoretical. For certain persons with low vision the results will not be as mathematically precise. However, the fact remains that the closer one gets to the chart, the smaller-size letter he or she is able to read.

"Legal Blindness" Defined

Some doctors vehemently reject the use of the word "blind" when talking about persons who are partially sighted. I understand and agree with this position, which emphasizes that a person who is partially sighted is not "blind." This perspective accentuates the fact that any remaining vision is useful. I also accentuate the positive view that persons with visual impairment still have useful vision, but I recognize the need to educate people as to the meaning of the word "blind."

The word "blind" may call to mind a person walking down the street with a white cane or a guide dog, but "blind" is a legal term. There are two ways a person can become "legally blind."

Loss of Visual Acuity

There are varying degrees of vision loss. Years ago, authorities arbitrarily drew a line: If one's visual acuity dropped below a certain level, he or she was declared blind. Since most people classified as "blind" enjoyed some remaining useful vision, the term "legally blind" evolved as a way of distinguishing them from the totally blind, who have little or no light perception.

Notice that the line drawn implied that such people's vision was nearly useless. Even today, this attitude persists and may explain why many doctors "write off" patients whose vision drops to this level.

At one time, states used different definitions of legal blindness. Some used a visual acuity of 20/400, while others used 20/200. Because the federal government pays 80 percent of rehabilitation costs for the blind, most states eventually adopted the federal standard of 20/200 so they could qualify for federal funds. Some states refer to legal blindness as "industrial blindness." This term also implies that vision below 20/200 is useless, in this case, for employment.

If the reader understands nothing in this book other than this one point, he has not wasted his reading time. Legal blindness does not mean a person is helpless or useless; it means he has a problem. With knowledge and help, that person can cope with the disability and can function with the vision he has left.

Field Loss

Visual acuity is only one measure of legal blindness. Retinitis pigmentosa and glaucoma can destroy peripheral vision, leaving only a 1-degree field of vision, which limits a person to seeing only straight ahead. (By contrast, a normally sighted person has a 180-degree field of vision.) The law states that a person whose visual field measures 20 degrees or less is legally blind regardless of her visual acuity. So, if someone's field of vision has been reduced to 1 degree, even if that 1 degree is 20/20, the person is considered legally blind.

How Test Charts Mislead

When I first began to lose vision and to take an interest in this subject, I encountered many people with a visual acuity of 20/200. But I never met anyone with a visual acuity of 20/150 or 20/175. This is because of a problem built into standard eye test charts.

Letter sizes on the typical eye test charts increase in units of 5 feet, jumping from 20, to 25, 30, 35, 40, and so on. After 80, the chart jumps 20 feet to 100. From there it jumps to 200, then to 400! Letter sizes larger than 400 are rarely found, except on special charts used in testing persons with subnormal vision.

Since the standard charts fail to discriminate between letter sizes, persons with a true visual acuity of 20/120, 20/150, or 20/180 are all diagnosed as 20/200. The doctor concludes, "This patient can't read the 100-size letter. The next size available is the 200-size, so that is how I must diagnose him." The same problem exists between 200 and 400.

Because of this inadequacy in the charts, persons with a visual acuity worse than 20/100 but better than 20/200 are all diagnosed as 20/200. Likewise, persons worse than 20/200 but better than 20/400 are all said to be 20/400.

A significant difference exists between the measurements of 20/105 and 20/200. Teachers are sometimes puzzled by the differences in performance of students who are all diagnosed with a visual acuity of 20/200. The student who is truly 20/105 will perform better than one who is 20/140. Both will outperform the student who is a true 20/200, yet all three are likely to have a doctor's report measuring their visual acuity as 20/200.

There is another variable related to performance and visual acuity. Tests can show that two people have the same visual acuity, yet they might perform differently. This introduces the subject of "functional vision." Functional vision relates to how well a person uses his or her residual vision. Time after time, I have met persons who say, "Your vision must be better than mine because I can't drive," or "I can't see TV," or "I can't read." When I've tested their visual acuity, I've often found that my vision is actually far worse. The difference is that I have learned to use my remaining vision better than they use theirs. My "better" performance can be attributed to vision rehabilitation — and enhancing performance through vision rehabilitation is what this book is all about.

Doctors may not be able to cure the disease that is destroying a person's vision, but the effects of the disease can be overcome or greatly minimized. These people can learn to function better, and the difference in performance is often dramatic. This is why a person's mindset and emotions play such an important role in vision rehabilitation. One's mindset and emotional state, as they relate to vision loss, can either block or boost all attempts at vision rehabilitation.

These facts are some of the most difficult for those with vision loss to accept. All their lives their eyes have worked. No special effort was needed to make them work. Then, when visual impairment occurred because of disease or accident, the situation changed. They must now learn to use their eyes in a new way. This book shows you how to use your remaining vision more effectively, but each person must incorporate these coping techniques into his or her own lifestyle.

Visual Impairment Defined

A person with a visual acuity of 20/120 can cope with his or her disability better than a person who measures 20/800. This is obvious even to a novice in the field. A person with a visual acuity of 20/60 has experienced significant loss, but he or she can still get a driver's license in many states. On a practical level, then, what do these visual acuity numbers mean?

There are numerous systems for classifying disability related to visual acuity. The visual disability scale that appears below is my own, and it is about as good, or inadequate, as any other.

First, several terms need clarification. **"Subnormal vision"** is defined by one's visual acuity after spectacles or contact lenses have been properly fitted. A person with a visual acuity of 20/400 corrected to 20/20 with glasses is not legally blind. The term **"legal blindness"** refers only to persons who cannot be corrected in both eyes using standard lenses; yet anyone not fully corrected to 20/20 has subnormal vision.

The terms **"object vision"** and **"travel vision"** need to be understood. "Object vision" describes the person with visual impairment who can see a brick house but not individual bricks. He can see a tree, but he cannot determine, in many cases, what kind of tree it is or distinguish individual leaves from a distance. He can see a person, but cannot determine whether that person is friend or stranger, even if he can determine the gender. In other words, the person can see enough to identify familiar objects, but he lacks definitive power. He cannot see details.

Early on, I lost the ability to see wrinkles on people's faces. In postgraduate school, one of my professors seemed about thirty-five or forty years old. She had to be around that age, I reasoned, because of her position as department head. A year later, she retired. She was sixty-five! Her face was wrinkled by age, but I couldn't see the wrinkles. I had lost definitive power.

"Travel vision" refers to how well a person can move around independently in an unfamiliar area without help from other people, a white cane, or a guide dog.

A Visual Disability Scale

20/20 — Normal vision.

20/25 to 20/65 — Subnormal vision, but not seriously impaired. Those below 20/45 have difficulty reading a newspaper, but most can hold it closer to their face and still read with good light. Many states will license people to drive with visual acuity as low as 20/60, but most such drivers will carry restricted licenses. Telescopic glasses allow all of this group to drive as long as their state permits it and if they do not also have serious field loss. These people have excellent object and travel vision, except for those who have lost considerable field vision as well as visual acuity.

20/70 — Mildly impaired. This is the point where people really begin to feel handicapped. Reading newspapers is very difficult without magnification, and most states refuse to license persons to drive with a visual acuity this low unless they are equipped with telescopic glasses. Object and travel vision are still excellent, except for those who have lost field vision as well.

20/75 to 20/200 — Moderately impaired. This group can still function as sighted in most regards with the use of low-vision aids. Object vision for this group is poorer, but it is still adequate for almost all activities. These people can see the car but may have trouble identifying its make and model. Recognizing friends may be difficult, but they see the person. Travel vision is still quite good unless there is also field vision loss.

Reading is the primary problem for this group, but good equipment and training eliminate this problem. I knew a young man on a high school football team who played wide receiver with a visual acuity in this range. He saw and caught the ball as well as other team members, but he had problems reading. People in this group can be equipped and trained to read using numerous low-vision aids. All members of this group should be able to drive with tele-scopic glasses unless there is also serious peripheral-vision loss, or other limiting factors.

Many rehabilitation agencies justify teaching Braille and the use of a white cane to people in this group who have a disease that may ultimately destroy all vision. While such an approach may make financial sense, I strongly support vision rehabilitation as the first step in training at this stage. If people in this group later lose even more vision and need blind rehabilitation, then I support giving them additional training at that point, when they will be more willing to accept it. People with functional vision are typically poor Braille and cane students. I believe that it is unnecessary, ridiculous, and a serious injustice to teach Braille to people in this group. They need to be equipped and taught to use the vision they have left. I have seen people in this group being taught Braille and the white cane wearing blindfolds. Nothing angers me more! They need vision rehabilitation, not blind rehabilitation.

20/200 to 20/800 — Seriously impaired, but still with travel vision and reduced but useful object vision. People in this group can read with low-vision aids of various kinds. In my opinion, those below 20/500 might consider learning Braille, but even then it certainly isn't mandatory. These people will not be able to drive, even with telescopic glasses. Object vision diminishes but is still useful. Travel vision is still adequate, although those at the lower end of the scale may sometimes trip over curbs. Crossing streets can be hazardous for people at the lower end of this scale because they cannot see distant oncoming cars.

I worked with a young woman at Baylor University in Waco, Texas, whose visual acuity was 20/800. She often developed "cabin fever" and wanted to get out of the house. She walked around the block, but dared not cross a street. She simply couldn't see oncoming cars. She was supplied an 8X handheld telescope, which improved her vision to 20/100 (800 divided by 8 — the scope's magnification level — equals 100). It gave her independent mobility in her neighborhood and on campus.

20/800 to 20/1200 — Severely impaired. At this level of visual acuity a person loses travel vision. People suffering a loss of peripheral vision may find a white cane useful or even necessary before this point is reached, but at this stage, use of the white cane becomes necessary, regardless of the cause of vision loss.

Some in this group are able to use very strong magnifiers to read large print. A +50 diopter lens ("diopter" — usually abbreviated as "D." — is the unit of measure of the strength of a lens) will give almost all in this group the ability to read textbook-size print. The reading aid of choice is the video visual aid (discussed in Chapter 22), which enables people in this group to read even small print. Object vision is poor, but any that remains is useful. Telescopic devices can aid in distance viewing.

20/1200 to 20/6000 — Very severely impaired. Many doctors reject the use of visual acuity figures this low. While it is true that letter sizes larger than 700 do not exist on test charts, there are mathematical equivalents. For example, 1/200 is the same as 20/4000 (remember that visual acuity is expressed like a fraction or ratio), which informally equates to the ability to count fingers at a distance of one foot. A visual acuity of 2/200, therefore, equals 20/2000; 4/200 equals 20/1000; and 2/600 (a letter size found on low-vision test charts) equals 20/6000. Doctors categorize this level as the ability to see a hand moving one foot away, without the ability to count fingers.

People in the 20/1200 to 20/6000 group are dependent on the white cane or a guide dog for independent mobility. A video visual aid for reading print is the aid of choice and the only aid that provides visual access to print. (The lowest visual acuity I have ever tested on a person who could still use a video visual aid was 1/700 or 20/14,000.) Voice synthesizers are available that convert print into speech. Persons in this group are legitimate users of such equipment, but such machines are beyond the scope of this book.

This group has little object vision, but as long as there is any light perception, that vision is useful. For example, a man walking down the street with his white cane sees two shadows ahead. He sees light between the two objects. He probably can't tell what the objects are, but he knows there is space enough between them for him to pass through.

Disability: Handicap or Challenge?

There are two dramatically different views of disability caused by visual impairment. One person might view it as a handicap. This person is likely to give up. God, nature, or fate has dealt him a bad hand and nothing can be done about it. Another might view the disability as a challenge, something to be resisted and overcome. This person will find a way to continue living life productively.

For those who find themselves tempted to see their disability as a handicap, let me recommend a book titled Challenged to Win, by Nancy K. Shugart.

I have known Ms. Shugart, a visually impaired music teacher in Austin, Texas, for more than twenty years. Her book tells how she dealt with macular degeneration and retinitis pigmentosa before age twenty and then diabetes later in life. It provides incentive and inspiration for anyone. Ms. Shugart founded Expect to Win Enterprises, a company working to inspire both children and adults to win the challenge of disability. The address of her organization appears in Appendix B.

Testing Your Visual Acuity

Among the persons in this country classified as blind or legally blind:

- ◆ 6 percent are totally blind, with no light perception;

- ◆ 19 percent have only minimal light perception;

- ◆ 75 percent have residual vision, almost all of whom are candidates for the use of low-vision aids and vision rehabilitation.

These figures surprise many people. Almost all of the money spent in past decades on rehabilitating the visually impaired was directed toward the needs of the totally blind. This is a classic example of the tail wagging the dog. The blind are not to blame for this nor should the legally blind hold any animosity toward them because of it, but it does explain why vision rehabilitation has lagged so far behind blind rehabilitation.

The percentages above need clarification. Many doctors do a very poor job of testing visual acuity below 20/100, especially if the patient is known to have one of the diseases discussed in this book. Ten years ago, I met a woman who had been told by her doctor that she was totally blind. She believed it. When I tested her visual acuity, I found it to be 20/800. If a doctor had prescribed glasses to correct her nearsightedness and astigmatism, her visual acuity would have tested even better.

Countless people have shown me doctors' reports diagnosing them with age-related macular degeneration and assigning them a visual acuity of 20/6000, or "the ability to see hand movements at one foot." I taught these people eccentric viewing (see Chapter 14) and then tested their visual acuity to find that, in fact, they were 20/200 or rarely lower than 20/240.

Thousands of persons, written off by doctors who say they have only minimal light perception (those in the 19 percent group), in fact have a testable visual acuity. Almost all can read print with a video visual aid, if not standard magnifiers. These facts indicate that the practices of modern eye care seriously need reexamination. Repeatedly, I have cautioned persons with partial vision not to trust the visual acuity assigned by a doctor unless the doctor is a low-vision specialist. The warning is applicable to those who have a visual acuity below 20/100.

So how can you feel more certain of your own visual acuity? Visual acuity is the product of two variables: letter size and distance. It is possible, therefore, to get a fairly accurate assessment of visual acuity if one of these variables is a given.

Appendix A shows test numbers 8 – 3 – 6. These numbers are the 100-foot size, meaning a person with normal vision can read them standing 100 feet from the chart. Those who would like to check their own visual acuity may do so by following the instructions below.

Set the chart from Appendix A in good light, and then find the most distant spot from the chart where you can still read all three of the numbers. Since you have seen the numbers, you must be honest about actually being able to read all of them rather than just remembering them.

(Note: For an accurate assessment, those who have lost central vision from macular problems must learn to use eccentric viewing before doing this test. See Chapter 14 for an explanation of eccentric viewing. Those who once wore distance glasses or contacts should wear them when doing this test, even if they help very little.)

Carefully measure (in feet) the farthest distance from the test chart where you can read all three of the numbers. Compare the findings with those in Table 1.1 to obtain a realistic measure of your true visual acuity.

Table 1.1 — Converting Feet to Visual Acuity

100 feet equals 20/20, normal vision

50 feet equals 20/40	25 feet equals 20/80
20 feet equals 20/100	18 feet equals 20/120
16 feet equals 20/140	14 feet equals 20/160
12 feet equals 20/180	10 feet equals 20/200
8 feet equals 20/240	6 feet equals 20/333
5 feet equals 20/400	4 feet equals 20/500
3 feet equals 20/650	2 feet equals 20/1000
1 foot equals 20/2000	½ foot equals 20/4000

These figures are valid only when test letters or numbers are the 100-foot size.

CHAPTER 2

Understanding the Eye

If you know how the eyes work, you will better understand the effects of disease on your vision. Knowledge is the first step in overcoming the consequences of disease.

The Eyeball's Shape

The normal eyeball is round. Irregularly shaped eyeballs cause the most common vision problems: nearsightedness and farsightedness.

Nearsightedness

Nearsightedness is caused by an eyeball that is too long from front to back. The clinical term for this condition is **myopia**. In myopia, the eyeball is so long that light from distant objects is brought to focus short of or on the "near" side of the retina, which lines the back of the eyeball (see Figure 2.1) — thus, the term "near-sighted." Light from near objects, on the other hand, is focused more sharply onto the retinal surface, so near objects appear in focus to the nearsighted viewer.

Research during the late 1920s showed that 30 percent of the U.S. population was nearsighted. Today the percentage is closer to 65. Some doctors blame the increase in nearsightedness on genetics. A more important factor may be that people today learn to see up close, and do not spend as much time learning to see at distance. Daniel Boone didn't spend much time keeping tax

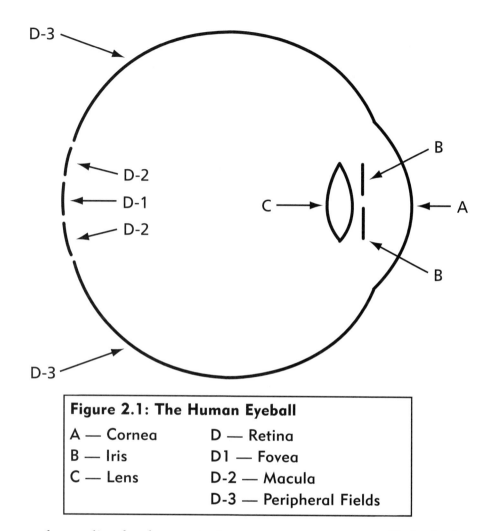

Figure 2.1: The Human Eyeball

A — Cornea   D — Retina
B — Iris   D1 — Fovea
C — Lens   D-2 — Macula
                    D-3 — Peripheral Fields

records, reading books, or staring at computer screens. He looked at distant objects. He watched for game to shoot while hunting or for dangers lurking while scouting. Today, from childhood onward, people engage in many more activities that require them to see up close. Modern humans learn to see better up close, while our fore-bears learned to see better at a distance.

As discussed above, a nearsighted person can see things better up close. His or her distance vision blurs. Spectacles or contact lenses can correct myopia, unless another complicating condition exists.

One form of nearsightedness deserves additional attention: **progressive myopia,** sometimes called **galloping myopia.** Galloping myopia, usually seen in teenagers, is characterized by rapid changes in the shape of the eyeball. The back of the eyeball expands, pushing the retina farther and farther from the lens and worsening the myopia. This situation can potentially produce an even more serious problem. The eyeball is fairly elastic and can expand somewhat without undue damage, but the retina is not as elastic. When the eyeball expands, the retina is stretched like a drumhead. It can tear or detach under such conditions. If it does not tear or detach, it may remain intact until a blow to the head or eye causes it to break loose.

People who are very nearsighted (requiring more than -5 D. lenses; see below for discussion of lenses) should avoid contact sports. As a minimal precaution, they should wear sports goggles while playing games where there exists a possibility of being hit in the eye. A detached retina is always a danger for sufferers of severe myopia.

Farsightedness

Farsightedness, or **hyperopia,** is caused by an eyeball that is too short. The eyeball tries to focus light onto the far side of, or beyond, the retina. The hyperopic person has trouble seeing up close. He sees distant objects more clearly. Farsightedness is not a major problem. Standard lenses will usually correct it.

Corrective lenses — eyeglasses or contact lenses — correct the problems caused by irregularly shaped eyeballs by bending, or refracting, light so that the focus falls on the surface of the retina, rather than in front of or behind it. People who are nearsighted are prescribed negative (-) lenses. People who are farsighted are prescribed positive (+) or magnifying lenses. Bifocal lenses are positive lenses added to a person's regular prescription. If a person's regular prescription is a negative lens, his bifocal lens will simply have less negative power. For example, a person with -6 diopter lenses who needs +5 diopters of magnification will have bifocal lenses that are -1 D. (-6 D. plus +5 D. equals -1 D). Those who require positive lenses to correct their refractive error will have even stronger bifocals. For example, a person with positive lenses of +2 D. who needs +5 D. in his bifocal lens will have +7 D. bifocals.

When a person develops a disease of the eye, the doctor might tell him, "Glasses won't help." This is because ordinary corrective lenses, for the most part, correct vision only when the problem is an improperly shaped eyeball. Standard lenses do not correct problems such as a retina that is being destroyed by disease.

Figure 2.1 is a drawing of the human eyeball as seen from the side. The drawing is not exact; it has been modified so readers with visual impairment can see it better. The letters and numbers on the drawing correspond to the parts of the eye described below.

A. The Cornea

The cornea is a tough membrane covering the front of the eyeball. It plays a role in focusing light onto the retina. The cornea is the only part of the eye that can be transplanted. Corneas obtained from donors are transplanted to the eyes of persons with corneas damaged by accident or disease.

Complete eyeballs cannot be transplanted, because the optic nerve that carries signals from the eye to the brain is unlike other nerves in the body. The optic nerve is actually part of the brain. It is the extension of the brain that goes out to the "light sensors" we call eyes. Since the optic nerve is part of the brain, surgeons must learn to transplant brains and spines before they have the technology to transplant eyeballs.

The cornea is made of very special tissue. It receives its nourishment from tears and from the aqueous humor (fluid) inside the eye and only indirectly from the circulatory system. All the cornea needs is oxygen. It absorbs oxygen from tears.

If a person's contact lenses do not fit correctly, he or she experiences a clouding of vision. This is because the contact lens is not permitting tears to circulate under it, and so the cornea is "starving" from lack of oxygen.

An imperfectly shaped cornea — one that is a little lopsided — causes astigmatism.

B. The Iris

The iris is the colored part of the eye. The hole in its center forms the pupil. The iris is like the diaphragm in a camera that can be changed to control how much light reaches the film. In the dark, the pupil opens wide. In bright light, the pupil gets smaller; that is, the iris closes, reducing the amount of light entering the eye.

When a person reaches age sixty-five or seventy-five, the muscles that open and close the iris often become stiff and unresponsive. At this age, the pupil may lose its ability to change size.

This explains why some older people have problems going from a brightly lit area into a dark room. The pupils are locked in a position that limits how much light can enter the eye, so they have problems seeing in dim light. This also explains why many older people become photophobic, or sensitive to light. The irises are locked in an open position, so too much light enters the eye.

When too much light enters the eye, a person is "blinded." His visual acuity drops dramatically. This is what happens to the albino who has a translucent iris that cannot control light entering the eye.

Traditionally, eye-care professionals give albinos opaque contact lenses with a clear section in the center. This gives them an artificial iris, and the clear center becomes the pupil. This procedure sometimes corrects their vision; often it does not. It often fails because albinos have too little pigmentation in the sclera, or the white of the eye. Light passes through this tissue as well.

Some doctors, understanding this, have made scleral contact lenses for albinos. Scleral lenses are large, covering the white of the eye as well as the cornea. Once the lenses are fitted, a specialist paints them to resemble natural eyeballs. For children, the improvement is sometimes dramatic. In adults, a learning process must occur before vision is significantly improved. More will be said about this learning process in Chapter 3, "How We See."

C. The Lens

The lens inside the eye focuses light onto the retina. Without this lens and its ability to focus light sharply, humans could not see clearly. The cornea provides 60 percent of the focus, and the lens provides 40 percent. The cornea provides general focus while the lens refines and sharpens the image.

A cataract is a cloudiness that has developed in the lens, obstructing the passage of light through the lens and obscuring vision. Cataract surgery in the past involved the removal of the clouded lens. People who have had the lens of the eye removed are said to be **aphakic.** The lens is composed of clear fluid inside a clear membrane called the "lens capsule." Today the more common practice in cataract surgery is to suck the cloudy fluid out of the lens capsule and replace it with a plastic intraocular lens that goes inside the capsule. See Chapter 8 for a more thorough discussion of cataract surgery.

As people grow older, the fluid in the lens turns yellow. Some doctors believe this is the beginning of cataracts. They see cataracts as an inevitable part of the aging process. All one has to do is live long enough, these doctors maintain, and cataracts will develop due to this yellowing of the lens. Other doctors see this yellowing simply as a part of the aging process, having nothing to do with cataracts.

The lens in the eye is a truly amazing organ. It instantly and automatically focuses light onto the retina whether the light comes from near or far. This may not sound so impressive until you realize that a lens must be thick in the middle to focus light from objects nearby. It must be thin in the middle to focus light from objects twenty feet or more away. This means that the lens changes shape instantly and automatically every time you look at an object at a distance different from the last object you looked at.

The lens can do this because, rather than being rigid, it is a clear capsule containing clear fluid. The lens assumes exactly the right thickness to focus on targets, no matter what the distance. It accomplishes this by means of muscles surrounding the capsule. When you look at distant objects, these muscles contract and stretch the lens until it is thin. When you look at something nearby, these muscles relax and allow the lens to grow thick in the center. In younger adults, the lens has the remarkable ability to focus from four inches to infinity.

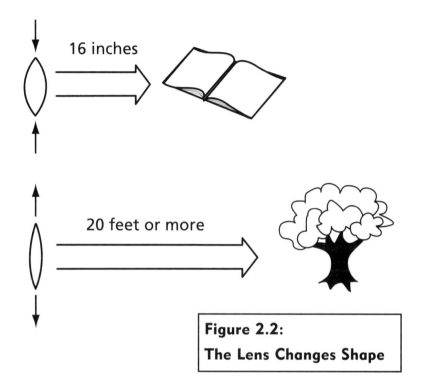

16 inches

20 feet or more

Figure 2.2:
The Lens Changes Shape

When humans reach the age of forty or so, the muscles around the lens have contracted and relaxed so many times that they begin to wear out. They stiffen and calcify, and eventually they no longer relax enough for the lens to focus on things up close. At this point, doctors prescribe bifocals, small positive lenses that help the natural lens to focus at reading distance. Doctors call this inability to focus naturally at reading distance the loss of "accommodation."

D. The Retina

The retina is a lining inside the eye covering the entire back half of the eyeball. There are several parts to the retina. The entire retina helps us to see, but each part performs a different function.

D-1. The Fovea

The fovea is a tiny spot on the retina directly behind the pupil. It measures 1.5 millimeters in diameter (less than one-sixteenth of an inch). The fovea provides sharp vision or 20/20 vision.

The field of vision the fovea provides is very small, about as wide as one finger when the hand is held out as far as one can reach. This simulates 1 degree of arc. By comparison, the compass has 360 degrees. There are 90 degrees of arc from north to east. There is only one degree of 20/20 vision in a normal eye. The rest of the retina cannot provide 20/20 vision.

D-2. The Macula

The macula is a small round spot on the retina that surrounds the fovea. It is sometimes called the "yellow spot." It measures about 4.5 millimeters in diameter (about three-sixteenths of an inch).

The macula (together with the fovea) provides 5 degrees of vision. The visual acuity provided by the macula, not counting the fovea, is from 20/40 (close to the fovea) to about 20/200 near its outer edge. To simulate how wide a visual field is provided by the macula, hold one hand out in front as far as possible. The macula and fovea together control an arc of vision as wide as the palm with the thumb held close beside it. This simulates a 5-degree field of view.

The macula is the part of the retina affected by macular degeneration. In this context, the fovea is part of the macula, so it is also affected by macular degeneration. When macular degeneration destroys the fovea and macula, this part of the retina no longer functions. Instead of fully functional retinal tissue, the person has a blind spot, called a **scotoma.**

For the patient with macular degeneration, the blind spot is a cone-shaped area. It appears as a spot less than two inches in diameter on targets sixteen inches away, such as the page of a book. On a target twenty feet away, the blind spot will appear as a circle four feet in diameter. On a target one block away, the blind spot will be as wide as five lanes of traffic.

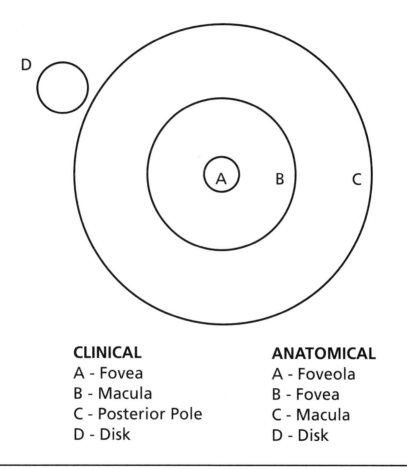

CLINICAL	ANATOMICAL
A - Fovea	A - Foveola
B - Macula	B - Fovea
C - Posterior Pole	C - Macula
D - Disk	D - Disk

Figure 2.3: The Surface of the Retina

Shows the relative position and size of the macula and fovea and their relationship to the disk. The disk is where the optic nerve attaches to the eye.

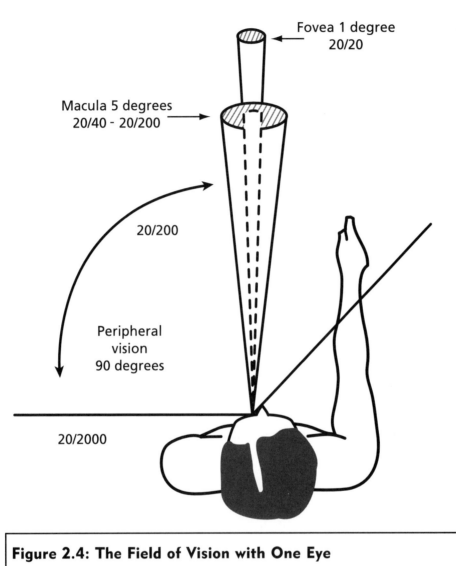

Fovea 1 degree
20/20

Macula 5 degrees
20/40 - 20/200

20/200

Peripheral
vision
90 degrees

20/2000

Figure 2.4: The Field of Vision with One Eye
Notice the field of view given by each part of the retina and
the range of visual accuity related to each part.

It is worth pointing out that doctors do not all mean the same
thing when they use the terms "macula" and "fovea." Doctors in a
clinical setting will use the terms to mean one thing, while doctors

in an educational setting or doctors speaking anatomically will mean something different.

Figure 2.3 illustrates how these terms are used differently under different circumstances. **This book uses only the clinical definitions of these terms.** The drawing shows the surface of the retina as a doctor might see it when he or she looks inside the eyeball through the pupil.

D-3. Peripheral Fields

The third part of the retina provides peripheral vision or side vision. Side vision is an imprecise term, because peripheral vision surrounds central vision, extending above and below it as well as to each side.

When persons with normal vision look straight ahead, they see things all the way around to their ears. Objects at the extremes of peripheral vision are not sharp, but they can still be seen. Peripheral vision provides object vision, but little definitive power. The visual acuity in peripheral fields ranges from about 20/200 (near the macula) to somewhere about 20/2000 straight out to the right or left.

Macular degeneration destroys only the macula and fovea, not the entire retina. Peripheral vision, therefore, is never affected by macular degeneration. This is why doctors tell patients with macular degeneration that they will never go completely blind. By contrast, retinitis pigmentosa and glaucoma destroy peripheral vision first, but also carry the potential of destroying the fovea and macula. People with these conditions risk losing their sight completely.

Figure 2.4 shows the field of vision with one eye as if you were on the ceiling looking down at this person's head. Notice the field of view given by each part of the retina and the range of visual acuity of each part. Notice how small an area of vision is controlled by the macula and fovea. Notice particularly how narrow our 20/20 vision is.

CHAPTER 3

How We See

Many people believe the eyes provide vision. This is only partially true. Actually, we see with our brains. The eyes detect light; that is all they do. Vision involves more than this.

Electrical Codes

When the eye senses light, it sends a coded, electronic signal to the brain. The brain must then interpret what the coded message means. Once it has translated the code, people see, but not until that time.

How does the eye sense light? The previous chapter began discussing the eye and how it works; however, the discussion was incomplete. The surface of the retina contains millions of light-sensing cells. They cover the surface in layers. Each of these light-sensing cells is photoelectric. That is, it is an electrical generator. When light strikes the cell, it generates a charge of electrical current that goes to the brain. What gets to the brain, then, is not an "image" of what is seen. Rather, it is a complex, coded, electronic signal. The brain must then identify, or translate, the code, and when it does, humans see.

These photoelectric, light-sensing cells are like switches. They have only two positions: on or off. Go back to that moment when as a child you first learned to identify certain kinds of trees. You looked at a spruce and someone told you, "This is a spruce." When you looked at the tree, light reflecting from the tree focused onto your retina, and certain light-sensing cells turned on; that is, they fired. They generated an electrical charge that went to your brain. Some light-sensing cells fired and some did not, so some cells were ON or "O" and some were OFF or "F." What went to your brain was a pattern or code of O's and F's.

The signal for "spruce" might look something like this: OOOFFFOOO. (This example is greatly simplified since only a few "cells" are shown, when in real life millions of cells would be involved.) In a compartment of your brain, you recorded that "OOOFFFOOO" meant "spruce." Later, you learned that "OOOFF-FOOOF" meant "Douglas fir," and "FOOOFFFOOO" meant "spiral pine." The code for each kind of tree registered in your memory.

Some time later you saw another spruce tree. Light-sensing cells sent the code "OOOFFFOOO" to the rear compartment of your brain. The computer in your memory bank functioned for a millisecond. When a match was found on file in your memory for the signal being received, you were able to "see." The computer then flashed a message to the frontal lobe of your brain: "You are seeing a spruce tree."

Vision as Memory

A baby comes into the world as a blank slate. He opens his eyes, and the eyes do their job, but there is no "vision" because the memory bank is empty. The infant has not yet learned to identify the millions of codes sent to the brain by the eyes. We all know that a baby doesn't focus his eyes for several months after birth. Why should he? His eyes are sending messages not yet understandable to the brain because it has no knowledge of these codes. The day will come, however, when the bottle that has been poked into the infant's mouth repeatedly for weeks will register in memory.

"Yesterday when I saw 'OFFOOF,' I got something to eat." Today the eye sends the message "OFFOOF," and the child remembers that this code means "bottle" or "nourishment." He finally "sees" or recognizes (which literally means "to know again") the bottle.

Seeing, therefore, is memory. People must learn how to see. They must learn all the specialized codes for every object in their environment. Seeing for adults is routine; they give it no thought. For infants, it is a learning process that continues for years.

Children who lose all vision before about age seven cannot visualize or conceptualize things described to them. Their visual memories have too little information to work with. If, however, they lose all vision after about age seven, their visual memory is large enough to support visualization and to understand descriptions of things they have never seen.

When disease destroys visual ability and reading becomes difficult and infrequent, people forget the code for words they have not seen in a long time. After about a year, they forget seldom-used words like "enhance" and "numb," to list only two examples. Different people lose different words. Reading ability may regress to the first- or second-grade level if one remains unable to read for about five years.

It can be painful to watch such people try to read. Anyone working in vision rehabilitation has helped patients regain reading ability who have not read for more than a year. They read along just fine until they come to a seldom-used word, and then they stop. They sit there staring at the word, embarrassed because they can't identify it. It may be a word they use in everyday speech, but they don't recognize it on paper, because they have forgotten the code for the word.

If this happens to you, spell the word aloud. This simple procedure is usually sufficient to recognize the word. Before reading further, look at the word again. Begin rebuilding the memory of how that word looks. Memorize the code!

For the visually impaired, there is another problem related to the role of memory in vision: the problem of diseases that destroy part of one's vision. As a consequence of such diseases, light-sensing cells in some part or parts of the retina are dead or no longer function. This means the eye has suddenly changed the code. When people with central vision loss from macular degeneration look at a spruce, their eyes may send the code "OOO — OOO" to the brain where it once sent "OOOFFFOOO." The eyes of those who have lost peripheral vision may send only " — FFF — ." This is not the same code that formerly meant spruce. The visual memory bank cannot find a match on file for the code currently being received from the eye. This explains the visual confusion and inability to identify familiar objects experienced by the visually impaired.

Even if a miracle happens and the disease stops destroying one's eyes, vision may become worse, **because the visually impaired forget how to see.** I say this not to frighten anyone, but to encourage readers to realize that, unless they do something to overcome the effects of the disease on visual memory, their situation will grow worse. Techniques presented in this book offer a good remedy for improving visual memory.

Two Kinds of Retinal Cells

There are two kinds of light-sensing cells on the surface of the retina: **cones** and **rods**. Cones, located primarily in the fovea and macula, provide sharp vision. Rods provide peripheral and night vision.

The outer edge of peripheral vision is provided exclusively by rods. The fovea, on the other hand, is made up exclusively of cones. Cones gradually diminish in number from the fovea out to the peripheral fields. Similarly, the number of rods increases from the macula out to the peripheral fields. This explains why central vision is sharp and peripheral vision is not. The two types of cells have different functions and capabilities.

Cones provide sharp vision. Since the fovea is 100 percent cones, it produces 20/20 vision. As the number of cones diminish toward peripheral fields, so does visual acuity. Cones require strong light before they will fire or function. In poor light, they cannot generate the electrical charge that goes to the brain.

On the other hand, rods cannot provide sharp vision. They simply do not possess this ability. They fire, however, when struck by the slightest amount of light.

Normally, people are not aware of this difference in the cells, but everyone has experienced their effects. Think about walking or driving down a street at night. While you are looking straight ahead, a dog jumps to the ground from someone's porch off to your right. Light reflecting from that dog, slight as it may be, enters the eye and focuses on the far outside edge of the retina. This area of the retina is covered with rods, which fire. Consequently, you see the motion of the dog. You may not have identified **what** moved, but you saw the movement.

When you detect movement, instinctively you turn your head and eyes to look directly at it. The dog is still there, but you can't see it! Why not? When you turn your head to look directly at the source of movement, the light reflecting off the dog now focuses onto the fovea rather than onto the outer part of the retina. Cones compose the fovea, and cones require more light to be activated. There isn't enough light reflecting off the dog and entering the eye for the cones to function, so you see nothing. You turn your head back to the front, wondering if you're going crazy. You must have imagined movement in that yard!

In fact, your eyes were working perfectly. They were performing exactly as they were designed to. Rods — which activate peripheral vision — fire with minimal light. Cones — which govern central sharp vision — require much more light.

Cones also provide color vision. People with macular disorders have color-perception problems. Technically, they may be color blind, but the problem is a difficulty in **perceiving** color, not an inability to **see** color. Typically, these people have trouble distinguishing between shades of pastel colors.

Concentration Rivets to the Point of Fixation

When we want to see something clearly, we look directly at it, so light is focused squarely onto the fovea. Consequently, our concentration fixes onto the relatively small area of vision provided by the fovea (a circle about ten inches wide on targets twenty feet away).

People concentrate so intently on what they see within this small circle of sharp vision that they are unaware of the blur they see in peripheral fields. I have asked people, "Look at a newspaper. How much of it can you see sharply at one time?" A person with normal vision looks at the paper. His eyes roam all over the page, and he answers, "I can see all of it sharply." Not so! He is able to read only a tiny circle about three-eighths of an inch in diameter at one time. He moves this sharp, foveal vision down the line of print or around on the page and says, "I can see it all sharply." The truth is, if he holds his eye and head perfectly still, he can see only four or five letters at a time, and he cannot read words on either side of this small area.

Speed-reading instructors tell students to learn to see more during each fixation. They say a person can learn to see the total width of a newspaper column. This is inaccurate. No one can teach the eye to do something it is physically incapable of. Speed-reading courses work, but not because students learn to see more at one time. What they learn is how to move the eyes more rapidly. Speed-readers still must scan the line of print four or five letters at a time, just like slow readers.

Only the fovea provides the ability to read small print. Of course, if larger print is used, some of the macula can read as well. The macula provides wider reading ability only when the print is Jaeger 4 or larger. To test near vision, doctors use a special test card containing paragraphs of material in different print sizes. Of the various print sizes on the card, the one known as "Jaeger 4" is the smallest size persons with a visual acuity of 20/40 can read without magnification. Recall that the visual acuity provided by the macula ranges from 20/40 to 20/200. The macula cannot read Jaeger 2 or 20/20 size print. The smallest it can read is Jaeger 4. Only the fovea can read Jaeger 2 (20/20) size print.

The Function of Peripheral Vision

A major function of peripheral vision is to detect motion. Peripheral vision senses light when the rest of the retina does not. When it does, humans have an automatic reflex that turns the eyes toward this detected motion. This brings their sharp, foveal vision into use.

Patients with macular degeneration, diabetic retinopathy, and (sometimes) cataracts must develop a special skill called eccentric viewing. Their central vision is gone, so they must depend on their peripheral vision. See Chapter 14 for a full discussion of how this is done. Before a person can learn to deliberately look away from what he wants to see, he must overcome the natural reflex to look directly at the target. Knowing about this reflex will help in the development of eccentric viewing skills.

Conscious Versus Unconscious Use of Vision

Based on what we've covered so far, it is obvious that seeing requires a great deal of mental energy. The person with normal vision expends this energy unconsciously, but the person with visual impairment must think about how he or she is using the eyes. One must "force" the eyes to obey, using conscious mental effort.

When a person with macular degeneration uses eccentric viewing, he or she forces the eyes to use peripheral vision instead of central vision. He or she must overcome the natural reflex to look directly at what he or she wants to see. This is distracting, and many people are unable to concentrate closely on another task while doing it.

When someone asks a person with macular degeneration to, for example, dial a phone number, she must concentrate on forcing her eyes to look **away** from the numbers. If she is given seven digits to dial, she may remember only three and need to ask for the last four to be repeated. Her conscious mind, engaged and preoccupied with seeing, may not concentrate well on the numbers recited to her. If she needs to devote conscious energy to making her eyes work efficiently, then doing so may distract from other conscious activity, such as remembering a phone number.

CHAPTER 4

Eye Fatigue and Pain[1]

Most eye diseases are not painful. (Glaucoma with a rapid onset is a notable exception.) However, while there may be no pain directly associated with the cause of vision loss, the eyes may hurt from the side effects of the disease. This chapter explains some situations that may cause the eyes to hurt. **Pain is often a warning that something is wrong.** If your eyes hurt, consult a doctor to make sure your condition isn't one that could be dangerous or destructive to residual vision.

Fatigue in the Nondominant Eye

One eye is always dominant; the other eye simply follows the lead of the dominant eye. People who are right-handed are likely to be right-eyed, and people who are left-handed tend to be left-eyed.

Many eye diseases begin their destructive work in one eye only. In other cases, one eye deteriorates more or faster than the other. For these reasons persons who lose vision usually enjoy better vision in one eye than the other. This better eye normally becomes dominant. If the disease begins in the dominant eye, patients are much more likely to detect the loss early. If it starts in the nondominant eye, they do not detect the loss as quickly.

In either case, the signal sent to the brain by the poorer eye is often rejected in favor of the clearer signal. When this happens, the poorer eye may quit working, and it may wander out or in, up or down from the point of fixation of the better eye. Once this happens, when patients look at something up close, like lighting a cigarette, the nondominant eye may try to match the fixation point of the better eye. This can cause a sharp pain in the eye that has been "off target." The muscles in the wandering eye are "out of shape"; they react like your legs would if you were to ride a bicycle for the first time in twenty years. They hurt!

Exercises such as the one described below may help to eliminate this type of pain, but you should increase the amount you exercise **gradually** — as you would increase the distance you ride a bicycle each day.

Sit more than twenty feet away from a visual target. Hold a pencil or other small object about ten inches in front of your eyes. Without moving your head, look at the pencil, then look at a distant object on the right. Look back at the pencil, then look at a distant object on the left. Repeat several times, all without moving your head. The objective in this exercise is to make the eyes move back and forth, thereby working the muscles that turn the eyes in their sockets. Do these exercises a few minutes each day to strengthen those flabby eye muscles that have gotten out of shape.

Eye Fatigue from Other Causes

There are several sets of muscles in the eye. The preceding section relates to the muscles that turn the eyes in their sockets. There are also muscles that change pupil size, and others that focus the eye at the proper distance. Once visual acuity drops so much that patients can't read, they tend to shift the eyes into neutral. They don't really make their eyes work.

Sometimes people deliberately do this, mistakenly believing they can save their residual vision. This is not true! **There is no**

way a person can damage his vision by using his eyes and the vision he has left.

If a person starts reading again with the help of a low-vision aid, a burden is placed on the eyes. They have to work, and various muscle groups may complain bitterly. You should increase your reading time gradually, just as you would begin a new exercise program. With persistent effort, the pain and fatigue will diminish in time.

Dry Eyes

Use of computers introduced a new problem, often called "computer eyes." People who worked with computers all day complained that their eyes hurt; they burned and felt tired. Researchers found that people who concentrated hard to read the letters on the computer screen were short-circuiting the body's unconscious blinking reflex.

Blinking lubricates the eyeball. Each time a person blinks, a new coating of tears moistens the eyeball. Heavy concentration can interrupt this reflex, so the eyeballs dry out. The eyes then feel rough, gritty, and painful.

This same short-circuiting effect can occur when patients first learn to read with a magnifier or a video visual aid. If you work with computers, or if you are learning to use visual aids, deliberately blink at the end of each line of print you read.

People over age forty whose eyes are drier than they used to be may profit from using artificial tears. Talk to your doctor. If he says artificial tears aren't necessary, try them anyway. The result is always soothing, and sometimes a dramatic improvement in vision occurs. Research indicates that dry eyes can reduce visual acuity to

20/200 when no other problem exists! Artificial tears are available without a prescription.

Ceiling fans can also dry the eyes, especially those of older people. Protect your eyes from the downdraft by wearing a brimmed hat, such as a baseball cap.

A person cannot damage his or her vision by using the eyes, nor can a person preserve the vision he or she has left by not using the eyes. If patients do not use their eyes, if they do not work them, if they do not continue to read using one of the aids this book describes, their functional vision will deteriorate. Seeing is memory! Recognizing words on the printed page is memory, and if people do not read by employing some type of aid, they forget how certain words look. If this happens, the patient can relearn what was lost, but it is much easier to **retain** reading ability than to **regain** it.

Part II

Other Things to Know

CHAPTER 5

Emotional Issues

One day, a man noticed that his vision was distorted: a telephone pole looked crooked; a windowsill looked wavy. This was the first sign that his vision was changing. Another person began noticing that she had difficulty seeing at night and that she failed to see movement to the side. Still another person noticed that her whole field of vision had become slightly blurred.

A time came at about age forty when the man could no longer read small print. He went to a doctor, who prescribed bifocals or reading glasses, which solved the problem. Now, however, the problem is different. Things have begun to appear darker, and a fog seems to linger, even indoors. The doctor says, "Glasses won't help." He explains that the patient has developed a disease of the eye.

The patient sits quietly, listening, but inside he screams in terror at the prospect of losing his vision. As the disease progresses, his vision deteriorates. The patient has trouble seeing small objects. He can't read the stock quotations in the newspaper; then he can't read the rest of the paper. Everything looks cloudy or blurred. A phone book produces only frustration, and he must depend on others to locate a number. He gives up driving because he no longer feels safe doing so. Depression sets in.

Depression

In this country, a person's ego or self-concept develops from the sum of what he or she can do, with emphasis on the word **do.** A person sees herself as worthwhile because she gets a promotion or successfully manages her family's finances. He can make enough money to afford a vacation. She can play a dynamite game of tennis. He can build a pleasing piece of furniture.

With diminished visual ability, most people can no longer do what they did previously. The result is that many begin to think of themselves as less worthy, less useful, less human than others — and depression ensues.

Doctors can treat depression. They can prescribe medication that works very well. But another way to conquer the depression resulting from eye disease is to learn how to overcome the consequences of eye disease.

This book offers answers, but the burden still rests squarely on you. You are the only one who can put what you learn in these pages into practice. Merely reading about the techniques of eccentric viewing, scanning, and getting close is not the same as mastering the techniques or incorporating them into your lifestyle.

To make these techniques work for you may require hours of study and effort. Those who master the techniques have the potential to reduce their disability to little more than a nuisance. By "nuisance," I mean that, even with reduced visual ability, you will be able to do most things people with normal vision can do. You will simply have to use an aid to do it.

I and others who have been lucky enough to find guidance and help are living proof that this is true. If a person's visual acuity is 20/800, he will be unable to do as much as the person who is 20/200. Nonetheless, he can still learn to use his vision more effectively. The only significant barrier to improvement is a resistance to learning something new.

Today, my corrected visual acuity is 20/240. Despite this loss of vision, I read anything I wish to read, no matter how small the print. Naturally, I must use an aid to help, but I can read! I have trouble locating a number in the phone book, but reading the number after finding it is no problem. I can sit twelve feet from a twenty-five-inch TV and see it well enough to enjoy a football game or a movie. I can't read the movie credits, but I can see the action.

I use a computer. This book was written using a standard IBM PC. Lastly, I drive wherever I want to go, in town or on the highway. When my visual acuity was 20/120, I drove at night on the highway and in unfamiliar cities. Since experiencing more deterioration, I have given up driving at night.

Can you function like this? It will depend on your visual acuity and on the type of vision loss you have experienced, but read on. Most patients can do much more than their family and even their doctors lead them to believe!

A note must be added here about driving. Few states will grant a driver's license to someone with a visual acuity below 20/200. The only reason I can drive with a visual acuity of 20/240 is because of my extensive experience. Using telescopic glasses, I have driven more than seven hundred thousand miles over the last twenty-nine years. In most cases, however, it is unrealistic to try to obtain a license with a true visual acuity below 20/200.

Note the word "true" in the statement above. Persons with partial vision are conditioned by their friends, relatives, and doctors, who tell them they can't possibly drive. Since pressure comes from all quarters, they believe it. They may accept that with aids they can read, but driving? No way!

Don't fall into this trap. Remember that a person who is visually impaired may have a visual acuity much better than what doctors have led him to believe. One's **true** visual acuity is the only limiting factor, if other variables support driving.

Independence Versus Dependence

A person with partial vision will always find things he or she cannot do as well as a person with normal vision. The best or most expensive aids cannot match the versatility and power of the human eye when it is undamaged by disease or accident.

Vision rehabilitation enables patients to improve their situation and to function better than before. They reclaim their independence and privacy as much as possible, given the degree of loss.

However, someone who has experienced vision loss will need help at times. To refuse help and try to go it alone is unrealistic and handicaps a person. On the other hand, depending on others for everything without doing what one can smacks of self-pity. Do not be afraid to ask for help when it is needed, but avoid dependence whenever possible. Dependence is deadly!

Grief

Grief is one of the most common emotional processes faced by persons with loss of vision. Grief is the process of mourning the loss of something valued or loved. The thing lost need not be a person; it might be a car, a favorite piece of jewelry, or any part of the body or its functions.

During grief, it is normal to feel anger. A wife loses her husband. She loved him very much, but she grows to resent him because he has left her alone. It is all part of the grieving process, and in time the hatred (grief) passes.

All who lose their vision experience grief, but people differ in the degree to which and length of time they grieve. Some people, angered by the disease that took their vision, build a compartment where they live separated from the disease and its horrors. They reconstruct the world as it was when they enjoyed normal vision, and they live in this fantasy creation. This world, this compartment in their thinking, is comfortable. They live there instead of facing and overcoming the reality of disability. When grief goes this far, it is time for someone in the family to take action and get professional help. The patient needs gentle encouragement to realize that grief is holding him or her back.

Secondary Gain

The psychological term "secondary gain" describes a personality pattern seen too often in disabled persons.

Grandpa Jones is a creature of habit. Every morning he gets up at seven. He goes outside to pick up his morning newspaper. He comes back into the house, gets a cup of coffee, sits down in his favorite chair, and reads the paper from front to back.

One morning he falls on ice and breaks his leg. He goes to the hospital and eventually leaves on crutches with his leg in a cast. The next morning, undaunted, he gets up, struggles to his feet, grabs his crutches, and heads for the front door. He is going after his newspaper, of course. His wife intercepts him. She takes him by the arm and tells him to sit down. She gets the newspaper for him. She even brings him his coffee. This is great, he realizes! He is eighty-seven, and the cold outside chills his bones. If Grandma Jones isn't careful, she may have a lifetime job.

It is bad to break a leg, but if that broken leg means someone gives us extra attention, something good results. This is secondary gain, and it can be deadly. It can block a person's efforts to improve their situation.

I knew a lady who harbored serious doubts about how well she had mothered her children. She felt she had done a poor job.

Proof of her failure came from the fact that her children never visited her, or at least they came less often than she liked.

When she developed macular degeneration and lost her central vision, her children responded well. Her son came by at least once a week to perform chores around the house. Her daughter came by several times a week to read her mail and write checks for her. Suddenly she had gained what she desired. Her disability had captured the concern and presence of her children.

At the insistence of her daughter the lady bought a video visual aid that allowed her to read and write again. Since she was now equipped to function independently, her children returned to the old pattern of visiting her once a month.

Eventually the lady sold her reading machine. She preferred the secondary gain of a closer relationship with her children to her increased independence.

Secondary gain can and often does prevent a person from overcoming a disability. It can disable one more than the disease itself. If a person with vision loss allows people to do things for him that he can do himself, this secondary gain may inhibit his recovery.

Everyone who experiences vision loss can benefit from the services of a psychologist or psychiatrist. These professionals can help patients deal with stress, depression, and other emotional issues. I have spent time in therapy and consider it one of the keys to my success in overcoming vision loss. Don't be stubborn or worry about what others might think. Get help! Emotional problems related to the loss of vision can prevent successful rehabilitation.

An alternative to seeing a psychologist is to join a local support group for people with a given disease. Such groups have become rather common in recent years. Ask your doctor or a counselor from the state commission for the blind if there is a group meeting in your area.

Progressive Loss of Vision

The person who loses vision quickly from an accident or from a disease that progresses rapidly is fortunate when compared to a person who loses vision slowly. If one's vision is suddenly lost and then stabilizes at a certain level, the patient can make the emotional adjustment and that's the end of it.

The person who loses vision a little at a time can have a far more difficult task. She loses part of her vision. She makes the emotional adjustment that allows her to go on with her life. The disease then raises its ugly head again and destroys more of her vision. The person suddenly realizes she can't do today what she was able to do a year ago. The emotional problems return, and she must deal with them again.

This may happen a dozen times, and it never becomes easier. If a person learns to cope with visual disability using techniques presented in this book, she has protection from the recurring emotional problems. If her vision worsens and the old aids no longer work, the patient knows that stronger aids are available, so she can continue to function despite additional loss.

Ego Defense Mechanisms

Most low-vision specialists fail to rehabilitate 35 to 50 percent of their patients. This is a sad but true statistic. Persons beginning vision rehabilitation can benefit from understanding why the failure rate is so high.

Earlier, this chapter discussed how in our society the human ego, or self-concept, is formed by the sum of things one can do. When visual impairment occurs, a gap develops between one's present ability and one's self-concept, which has always been based on what the person could do before losing vision.

The difference between how one formerly viewed oneself and the present reality puts the ego, or self-concept, under intense pressure. The conflict between the two is obvious. The human mind will not tolerate such a conflict, so it often develops an "ego defense mechanism" to reduce the pressure. Ego defense mechanisms are like the shock absorbers on a car. Shock absorbers protect passengers from the bumps in the road. Ego defense mechanisms protect people from the horrors of visual disability.

Psychologists have identified many different ego defense mechanisms. Some of the most common are repression, intellectualization, projection, and denial. My experience indicates that persons with visual impairment develop denial as the most common way of protecting the ego. With denial, the patient might openly talk about the disability, but deep down, at the subconscious level, he actually denies that things are any different now that visual disability has occurred.

Consider the following scenario. A person has developed denial as a means of protecting his ego from the reality of visual impairment. A low-vision specialist fits this patient with a pair of +20 diopter reading glasses. A +20 diopter lens requires reading material to be held exactly two inches in front of the lens for it to be in focus. As long as he is in denial, the patient will not use that pair of glasses. Why? Because a person with normal vision doesn't read like that! A person with normal vision holds the paper sixteen inches away, not two inches. The patient is emotionally denying his disability. He rejects the glasses. Before he can use the glasses or any other visual aid, of course, he must admit that he is disabled. So he makes excuses for why he doesn't use them: "They make my eyes hurt." "I can't see anything with them anyway." "They make me dizzy."

If after reading this book and consulting a low-vision specialist, the reader remains unable or unwilling to cope successfully with vision loss, emotional issues such as denial, grief, or secondary gain may be the cause. Such readers should definitely seek help, from either a psychologist or a self-help group. Persons with low vision **can** overcome or greatly diminish the consequences of visual impairment!

CHAPTER 6

Doctors

There are several specialties involved in eye care. Each concentrates on a specific area of expertise. Knowing what each kind of doctor does will help patients find the assistance they need.

Ophthalmologists

An ophthalmologist is a medical doctor who specializes in the treatment of the human eye. He or she has studied disease, medicine, and surgery related to the eye. Many people assume that such doctors have also studied vision rehabilitation. Such an assumption leads to trouble. Very few ophthalmologists study vision rehabilitation, so they can only help to remedy low vision if medicine or surgery will correct the problem.

    We humans tend to place doctors on pedestals or to make deities of them, but such an attitude does both doctors and patients an injustice. Doctors are human, subject to the same limitations as the rest of us. They are not gods. Think of a mechanic who has learned everything about car engines. If a car breaks down, the mechanic can fix it, but this doesn't mean the mechanic can drive the car. These are two different skills, and one does not ensure knowledge of the other. The ophthalmologist is like the mechanic. He or she studies the inner workings of the eye and can do many things for patients when things go wrong. Despite this, the average ophthalmologist knows little about subnormal vision and is not trained in vision rehabilitation.

If an ophthalmologist reads this book, he or she may pause after each chapter and be able to say truthfully, "I knew that." Still, the average ophthalmologist has not put the coping techniques presented here into a package or program designed to help the visually impaired.

Ophthalmologists often fail to recognize fully the benefits of the techniques discussed in this book. They know that light helps, for example, but they really aren't sure how much. They have seen patients with macular degeneration use eccentric viewing, so they know this skill exists, but they do not realize its full value.

Furthermore, many ophthalmologists have trouble believing that valid ways exist to help the visually impaired. If such methods exist, why didn't they learn about them in school?

A low-vision patient once insisted on help from his ophthalmologist. The doctor, under pressure, said, "You might see Dr. Swick. He has a hobby of working with low-vision aids." This attitude is unfortunately all too common. Many ophthalmologists see themselves vested with scientific knowledge; others merely play at the game. In fact, working with low-vision patients is an established science, not a hobby! Dr. William Feinbloom introduced the glasses I use for driving in 1926, decades ago, yet most ophthalmologists I've encountered are unaware that such glasses exist.

Consult an ophthalmologist for the problems they are trained to treat. Be cautious when they give advice or opinions related to subnormal vision or vision rehabilitation that don't require surgery or medication!

Optometrists

An optometrist is a person who has studied optics for four years. The optometrist's job is to fit glasses. He or she is trained to **detect** the symptoms of eye disease, but not to **treat** them. And just like the ophthalmologist, the optometrist may know little about vision rehabilitation.

Things are improving in this area. In recent years, schools of optometry have added low-vision study to their curricula. A given optometrist may choose not to work in this field, but he or she is more likely to know about low-vision work and to refer patients to someone who does.

Much overlap exists in the practice of optometry and ophthalmology. Many ophthalmologists fit glasses, and many optometrists check the eyes for disease. There is competition between these professions. Just as physicians and chiropractors sometimes fight for the same patients, so do optometrists and ophthalmologists. For this reason, ophthalmologists rarely refer patients to optometrists — and most, but not all, low-vision specialists are optometrists.

Because of the rivalry between these two professions, patients who go to an ophthalmologist for help when they develop an eye disease may find a dead-end street. If the ophthalmologist is unable to help by prescribing surgery or medicine, he or she may fail to refer patients to a low-vision specialist who is an optometrist. Optometrists also have a poor track record of referring patients to other optometrists who specialize in low-vision services. Referring patients to another doctor means a loss in patient load, which means less income.

Low-Vision Specialists

The third type of eye doctor is a low-vision specialist. This is the doctor who can do more for the visually impaired than anyone else when it comes to coping with vision loss that is unresponsive to medication or surgery. A low-vision specialist may be an ophthalmologist or an optometrist, but his or her specialty is to equip and train the visually impaired to function as sighted, using the vision they have left.

A low-vision patient is defined as one whose vision cannot be corrected with ordinary spectacles. Fourteen ophthalmologists told me there was no way they could give me the ability to read, drive, or watch TV from across the room. A similar number of optometrists gave the same verdict. When I met my first low-vision specialist, he didn't tell me the same bad news. He simply began equipping me to function sighted with the vision I had left.

The low-vision specialist equips a patient with hand magnifiers or magnifying spectacles that allow the patient to read print, including the gauges or dials on shop equipment and kitchen appliances. He or she equips a person with handheld telescopic devices or telescopes mounted in glasses that allow the patient to see more detail when viewing distant objects. If the doctor is really good, he or she will do much to neutralize some of the emotional problems that are blocking the patient's adjustment to functioning better. The specialist teaches skills like scanning and eccentric viewing that improve functional ability. In short, he or she teaches much of what is in this book.

I am not the founder or inventor of the techniques discussed in this book. They go back farther than my seventy-one years. I have simply compiled this information into one resource so that others like myself may find help.

If a person studies this book, does he or she also need to consult a low-vision specialist? Absolutely! This book expands a patient's idea of what is possible. It describes the skills he or she needs to master, but the low-vision specialist makes the possibilities in this book become reality. This book tells the story of vision rehabilitation and supplements what low-vision specialists do, but the low-vision specialist is the action figure who makes it happen.

Let me explain. Low-vision aids do exist that a person can select for himself or herself, and this book contains a chapter on how to compute the optical power one needs. When following the do-it-yourself route, however, exercise caution, because pitfalls exist when buying aids. For example, manufacturers frequently rate the power of their lenses incorrectly. If a person trusts the manufacturer's rating, he or she may be in for a disappointment that leads him or her to conclude, "I tried magnifiers, and they don't work for me." To use another example, a handheld magnifier — even one of proper power — may not be the best aid for an older person who is unable to hold it steady. He or she may need a "stand" magnifier that sits on the material being read instead of being held above it. The low-vision specialist helps people avoid these mistakes.

What Makes a "Good" Low-Vision Specialist?

All doctors are not equally competent — a truth that also applies to low-vision specialists. There is a great deal of variance in their performance. I have had the pleasure of knowing the best, and I have known some who were very poor.

How can the visually impaired locate a good low-vision specialist? I can name good low-vision specialists I have met, but I do not know doctors in all areas of the country. The best I can do is to give guidelines. You must then evaluate the performance of your own doctor. One of the purposes of this book is to empower the visually impaired to determine for themselves whether a doctor is doing a good job.

I asked my friend, Don Swick, O.D., of El Paso, Texas, to write a few paragraphs about his experience as a low-vision specialist. He has since passed away, but his insights provide a good summary of the different approaches taken by doctors who are low-vision specialists. His comments can help you distinguish between the truly effective low-vision specialist and one who is less helpful.

When I first began seeing low-vision patients, I found that measuring the best acuity and determining the theoretical magnification needed were not always enough to produce a well-cared-for patient. I learned that many factors control the outcome of the rehabilitation.

In fact, the definition of "low-vision rehabilitation" is: Multidisciplinary vision care preceding blind training of the visually impaired to obtain maximum visual independence and social adjustment.

In simpler language, this means: (1) the doctor must take the **whole** patient into consideration; (2) the doctor must help the patient regain as much independence as possible; and (3) the doctor must help the patient readjust to life and to his social situation under these new circumstances.

To learn how to meet these high standards, I took time out of my office practice and visited the best low-vision clinics and doctors. I picked their brains and watched them at work. This took me from New York to Los Angeles.

I found that there were doctors who thought that anything they prescribed had to be cheap and inconspicuous. They encouraged the patient to think this way.

Many doctors had an **assistant** interview the patient for case history and for the patient's expectations and wants. Many doctors had an **assistant** dispense aids and train the patient to use them. I observed that this did not result in a properly cared-for patient or a proper doctor-patient rapport.

I found doctors who sent patients home with glasses and systems to "try." Vision rehabilitation cannot be accomplished this way.

Professional care requires the doctor to become very involved. Returning to my own practice, I began requiring that the patient's next of kin be present, to observe the patient perform and to listen to me talk to the patient. I spent a lot of time discussing the condition of the vision and discussing what could be accomplished, along with how and why certain treatments would or would not work. As I examined and evaluated different optical systems and glasses, I trained the patient in their proper use and carefully explained the reasons behind these guidelines.

For the low-vision specialist to prescribe properly and train properly, he must do the counseling and train the patient himself. I observed the patient and the next of kin for problems that might affect the treatment's effectiveness, such as:

1. Hysteria and/or despondency

2. Emotional instability

3. The patient's expectations

4. The patient's previous advice from doctors, family, and agencies for the blind

5. The patient's previous experience

6. Expectations of the next of kin

Training the patient how to use the glasses or systems before measuring visual acuity is called "maximum proficiency evaluation." Following this procedure is essential for effective treatment, because when patients are taught skills such as eccentric viewing and are trained on the proper equipment **before** being tested, their true visual acuity can be measured.

In my experience, these methods taken together add up to a complete system of addressing all the needs of the low-vision patient.

Don Swick, O.D., Low-Vision Specialist

Let me add a postscript to Dr. Swick's comments. My first appointment with Dr. Swick lasted three hours. During this period he took a personal history, explored my needs and desires, diagnosed my condition, and tested various aids. When the aids he prescribed arrived at his office, I returned for another three-hour session, during which he trained me to use them. And after those first two appointments, I saw Dr. Swick many more times.

Finding a Low-Vision Specialist

Each state has a commission for the blind. In some states, this agency is called "visual services," a subdivision of the state department of rehabilitation. Call your local office and ask to speak to a counselor. Ask whom the agency recommends for low-vision services. Get the names of as many doctors as possible.

Call the American Foundation for the Blind, the American Academy of Ophthalmology, the American Academy of Optometry, or the American Optometric Association. Their telephone numbers are listed in Appendix B. These organizations maintain a list of low-vision specialists all over the United States.

Be reminded that not all doctors are equally qualified or motivated, even those whose names you secure from one of these professional organizations. As an example, I obtained the name of a doctor who is in my hometown from one of these organizations' lists. I found that he gives eye exercises and calls this low-vision work. If you are dissatisfied with the performance of one doctor, see another. If you consult with two or three and your results are still disappointing, reread the chapter on emotional issues and consider consulting a psychologist. The problem may lie in your own unresolved emotional blockages.

When considering a low-vision specialist, ask the receptionist or office assistant the following questions:

◆ Does the doctor take the patient's case history, or does an assistant do this?

◆ Does the doctor routinely lend aids to patients to take home and try?

◆ Does the doctor train the patient in the use of the aids he/she prescribes, or does an assistant do this?

In my experience, a better doctor-patient relationship is developed when the doctor himself or herself takes case histories and trains the patient to use aids, rather than relying on assistants to perform these tasks. By being intimately involved, the doctor remains in close contact with the patient's needs and progress. Having made this distinction, I must state that I know of good low-vision clinics that use assistants extensively. These are not meant to be hard and fast rules, only factors that must be computed into the equation when selecting a doctor.

The practice of lending aids to patients to take home and "try" appears to be a good idea on the surface. However, contrast this patient selection of aids to the doctor who carefully tests several lens systems and then prescribes one over another because it works better based on scientific tests. A patient's choice of aids is too often influenced by personal and emotional factors having little or nothing to do with vision.

CHAPTER 7

Perks and Privileges

Many people will find it surprising to learn that there are perks and privileges associated with being visually impaired. Believe it or not, this population does enjoy privileges not available to the normally sighted. A friend who is totally blind once commented, "Even a blind squirrel finds a nut occasionally."

Talking Books

The Talking Book Program, funded by the Library of Congress, lends recorded books and magazines to the blind and visually impaired. This service is free of charge. It is executed by state personnel who are usually but not always located in the state library. (Normally the library for the blind is part of the state library, located in the state capital.)

The books come on special audiocassette tapes, and the cassette player required to play the tapes is also provided, because ordinary tape recorders will not play these recordings. They are recorded at half of normal playback speed on four tracks per cassette instead of the normal two. Patrons can return the books to the library via the U.S. Postal Service's program called "Free Matter for the Blind," so even the postage is free.

These talking books are recorded by excellent professional readers, who often use different voices or inflections for each character. Almost any book you might desire is available. Patrons may make their selections from a catalog, or the state library for the blind can select the books from a profile prepared by the reader. The profile indicates what kind of reading the subscriber enjoys. Application forms are available from local public libraries or from the local offices of the state commission for the blind (called "visual services" in some states).

The Talking Book Program includes both fiction and nonfiction books, but it does not include textbooks. A different organization specializes in educational books. Refer to Chapter 33, "Education."

Free Matter for the Blind and Handicapped

People who are legally blind or otherwise handicapped so they cannot read have access to free mail service from the U.S. Postal Service (with certain restrictions, of course). The visually impaired may mail letters postage-free, if they are written in large print. The print must be fourteen-point type or larger, which is two to three times larger than standard typewriter print. Large handwriting should be acceptable as well. Place the letter in an envelope, but do not seal it. Tuck the flap inside the envelope and write the words "Free Matter for the Blind and Handicapped" where the stamp is usually placed. Do not include any standard-size printed material with the letter.

Postal regulations require all users of this service to be registered at the post office. You may register by sending a letter to your local postmaster, asking that your name be added to the list. Enclose a doctor's statement confirming that you cannot read standard print.

I use this privilege at times, so on my computer I prepared adhesive labels with this wording to use in place of postage stamps.

If you don't have access to a computer, you can order these stickers from businesses that print adhesive return-address labels.

This mailing privilege goes beyond personal letters. It includes the shipment of large-print books, supplies, and equipment used by the visually impaired. Talking-book machines, for example, are mailed as "Free Matter." Whereas letters must be left unsealed, supplies, equipment, and books may be placed in packages and properly sealed.

This free service applies only to mail delivered within the United States.

Free Directory Assistance

At one time, telephone companies provided free directory assistance. Today, people who are normally sighted must pay for this service. The visually impaired, however, may obtain free directory assistance from most (if not all) local phone providers and from AT&T by registering with these companies as a person who is legally blind. Once again, the letter sent to request this service must be confirmed by a doctor's statement. This privilege applies only to calls made from one designated phone number in the home.

Free Tuition

Texas and some other states allow visually impaired residents to attend state universities tuition-free (not including room and board). Contact the state commission for the blind (called "visual services" in some states) for more information about this privilege.

Gifted-Child Programs

In 1957, the Russians were the first to orbit a satellite around the earth. A great clamor arose in the United States following this event. "How can the Russians beat us into space? If they can do that, they can threaten us with atomic weapons. We need more and better scientists, and we need them now!" These were the Cold War years, and the country panicked.

The American educational system came under scrutiny. The United States had developed a great educational system for the masses, but it failed to nurture students with exceptional intelligence or talent. So-called "gifted-child" programs grew out of this furor. The programs vary from region to region, but they all rush gifted students through school faster than average ones.

I used one of these programs to obtain my doctoral degree. Since my vision was deteriorating, the university allowed me to enroll in the accelerated gifted-child program under the hopes that I could complete my degree before my vision became worse. The program I used allowed me to proceed immediately from the masters to the doctoral program without a work period between.

If one's vision is stable, such a program may not be appropriate. However, if one's vision is still deteriorating, a gifted-child program or one similar might save considerable time. Talk to university administration officials — such as a department head or the dean of students — about any accelerated programs available for the visually impaired. You do not need a superior IQ to qualify for these programs.

Descriptive Video Programs

A new service aids persons whose poor vision prevents them from enjoying television viewing. With the addition of a special "black box" that costs about $50, the viewer hears a second soundtrack describing what is happening onscreen as he watches and listens to the program.

Descriptive video programming may not yet be available everywhere. Call your local public broadcasting station for more information about this service.

More Perks and Privileges

Permits are available that allow the disabled to use handicapped parking spaces. I personally believe that the visually impaired should use this perk only if they are dependent upon a white cane for mobility. Handicapped parking, in my opinion, is for people with mobility problems.

Other perks for the blind are available, but low-vision patients may not appear sufficiently handicapped to qualify for them. Some of these benefits include free admission to movies and free passes on public transportation such as trains and buses.

Part III

Major Causes of Vision Loss

CHAPTER 8

Cataracts

An early symptom of cataracts is seeing halos around lights at night. This can also occur when a person develops glaucoma. Delay in seeing an ophthalmologist is **not** critical if cataracts are causing the halos, but if glaucoma is causing the halos, it is imperative to seek help immediately. Even a delay of hours can make a difference. **If you see halos around lights at night, call an ophthalmologist right away, describe your symptoms to the office assistant, and ask for an immediate appointment.** A well-trained assistant will understand the danger and arrange for you to see the doctor quickly. If you are given an appointment several weeks or even days in the future, protest and demand to be seen immediately.

A cataract is a clouding of the lens inside the eye that obstructs the passage of light through the lens and obscures vision. What causes the lens to become cloudy? Science does not have a definitive answer to this question, but many doctors believe poor nutrition plays a role. Research also indicates that persons who wear hats and sunglasses suffer a lower incidence of cataracts than those who do not. Infrared or ultraviolet light from the sun apparently plays a role in the development of cataracts.

Cataracts generally destroy both central and peripheral vision. Figure 8.1 illustrates loss of vision from cataracts. Cataracts may develop as a gradual, uniform clouding of the whole lens, or the clouding may be dense in one area of the lens and gradually

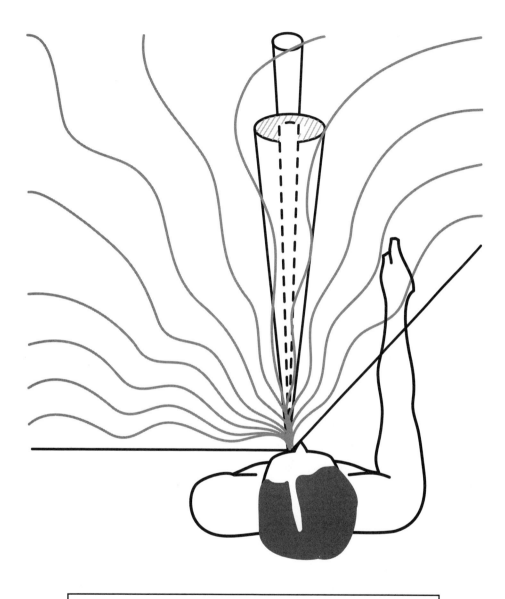

Figure 8.1: Vision Loss Caused by Cataracts
The wavy lines represent blurred, foggy vision.

spread to the rest of the lens. The rate of deterioration is always unpredictable.

The degree of density of cataracts varies widely. If left untreated, cataracts can become so dense that the person is virtually blind, with little light perception.

Cataract surgery involves the removal of the cloudy lens. But removing the lens deprives the eye of an important function: there remains no way to focus light onto the retina. In years past, and occasionally now, following cataract surgery the doctor would prescribe very strong positive lenses (spectacles or contact lenses) that focused light directly onto the retina from outside the eyeball. Today, however, the most common approach to replacing the cloudy lens removed during cataract surgery is to implant a plastic lens inside the eye.

During the 1960s, cataract surgery was a gory, time-consuming procedure. Patients had to remain in the hospital for days, their heads blocked with sandbags so they couldn't be turned.

The intraocular lens implant, developed during the 1970s, is now the preferred method. Initially, doctors suspended lens implants over the pupil with a hook-and-eye arrangement. "Eyes" on the lens and "hooks" attached to the iris suspended the lens over the pupil. This worked well until the patient sneezed hard and one of the hooks came loose! Later, doctors sewed the plastic lens to the iris, covering the pupil.

Today, new technology replaces these earlier implant techniques. The lens inside the eye consists of a clear fluid in a clear sac or capsule. The surgeon removes the cloudy fluid and places the plastic lens inside the sac. Intraocular lens implants generally provide a visual acuity of 20/20 to 20/40, but the eye loses some of its versatility. The plastic lens cannot change shape as the human lens did, so glasses are required for reading. The implanted lens is for distance viewing.

Before the days of intraocular implants, doctors often postponed surgery until the cataract became "ripe." This is an archaic expression no longer used by doctors operating with the new lens-implant technology. Prior to lens implants, doctors removed both the lens fluid and the capsule or sac containing it. As the cataract matured, the whole mass became hard, making it easier to remove both the fluid and the sac at the same time. A cataract that was not ripe was one that had not yet grown hard enough to be removed intact. Since surgeons today remove only the fluid inside the capsule, they do surgery before this hardening occurs.

Cataract surgery is so common and the procedure so simple that surgeons often perform it in a surgery center in their offices on an outpatient basis. Only occasionally do patients need hospitalization.

When Should Cataracts Be Removed?

This is a question only the patient can answer. I have listed guidelines below, but they are strictly my personal opinion. Each patient with cataracts must evaluate his or her own situation.

Cataract surgery is about as safe as any surgery performed, but no one can claim it is risk-free. Cataract surgery carries a failure rate of about 5 percent. Even if the surgery goes well, the patient can die from the anesthesia, or develop a staph infection immune to antibiotics. These are only two of the things that can go wrong; many more exist. Any surgery involves risks.

If I ever develop cataracts, I plan to follow these guidelines:

1. I will schedule cataract surgery when the cataracts begin to interfere with my lifestyle.

2. I will schedule surgery to remove the cataract from only the eye that provides the poorer vision. If all goes well, I will then schedule surgery on the other eye. If things do not go well with the first eye, I will delay surgery on the other eye as long as possible.

You are the only person who can decide when it is time to take the risks of surgery, but these guidelines may help.

CHAPTER 9

Diabetic Retinopathy

I had a professor in graduate school who required all his students
to read five professional journal articles each week and report on
them. Since I had a keen interest in vision loss, I did most of my
reading in journals devoted to that subject. One week, I reported
on a study of diabetic retinopathy. The study showed that persons
afflicted with diabetes developed retinopathy approximately fifteen
years after the onset of the disease, no matter how well the
diabetes was controlled.

I turned in my report, and that same day the professor
announced that he had been diagnosed with diabetes. If he read
my report, it was a startling way for him to learn what he faced.

Diabetes, the sugar disease, afflicts eleven million persons in
the United States. Fifty percent of them have or will develop
retinopathy ten to fifteen years after its onset. Because it strikes all
ages, diabetes is the leading cause of vision loss in the United
States, but new technology is reducing its impact.

Diabetes develops when the pancreas fails to produce enough
insulin to process the sugar needed to sustain life. Excessive
glucose (blood sugar) in the veins destroys blood vessels. Parts of
the body containing a high concentration of blood vessels, like the
liver, kidneys, and retina, suffer damage, or sometimes destruction.

Diabetic retinopathy is a cyclic disease. Excessive glucose
destroys some of the very small blood vessels in and beneath the
retina. This causes scar tissue to form. New blood vessels grow

through the scar tissue. Eventually they also deteriorate, creating more scar tissue. Scarring creates a blind spot, or scotoma. When this occurs in the macula, as it often does, visual acuity can drop quickly. However, the scar tissue can develop anywhere on the retina.

Diabetic retinopathy can affect both central and peripheral vision. Figure 9.1 illustrates a typical pattern of vision loss from diabetes. The illustration shows loss in part of the macula and loss in peripheral fields. Notice that the blind spots are shown in black, but the patient does not see black in these areas. The black simply indicates an area where the person has no vision.

Two Kinds of Diabetes

There are two kinds of diabetes: diabetes insipidus, caused by a problem with the pituitary gland, and diabetes mellitus, the more common and dangerous form. The two are unrelated, but both cause the patient to be thirsty all the time and to urinate a lot. The second type causes problems with the eyes.

Diabetes mellitus occurs in two forms: insulin-dependent (also called type 1) diabetes and noninsulin-dependent (also called type 2) diabetes.

Noninsulin-dependent diabetes, usually striking in adulthood and associated with obesity, is the less dangerous of the two. Diet and exercise will often control it without medication. Persons with insulin-dependent diabetes, on the other hand, should exercise only under strict supervision of their doctors.

Diabetes causes two types of retinopathy. The first, called background retinopathy, occurs as the first stage of retinopathy. As a rule, these patients do not face blindness or even severe visual problems. Eighty percent of these patients do not progress to the second stage.

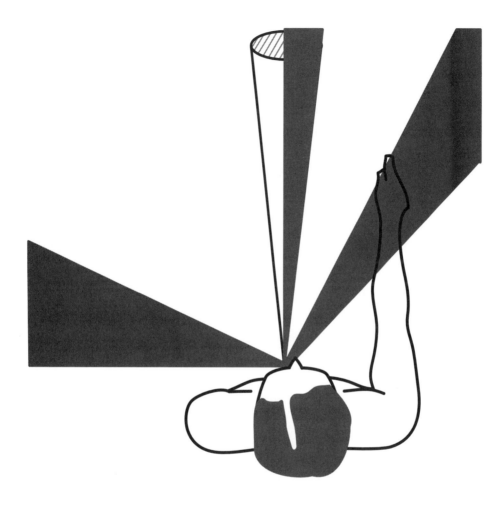

Figure 9.1: Typical Pattern of Vision Loss from Diabetes
Black areas represent blind spots.

Proliferative retinopathy, the second stage, is far more destructive than the background type. The effect on the retina is the same. The two types differ only in degree.

Treatment

The primary treatment for retinopathy today is treatment of the diabetes that causes it. The best thing diabetics can do for their eyes is watch their weight, exercise (under the care of a physician if they are insulin-dependent, excessively overweight, or new to exercise), take medication as prescribed, and avoid sugary foods.

The argon laser is an effective tool used today to slow or stop deterioration of the retina caused by diabetes, although it is not understood precisely why this treatment works. Doctors aim the laser at the deteriorating blood vessels on the retina. Laser treatments are not used if the deterioration occurs in the macula. The laser kills retinal cells wherever it is applied, so using it in the macula would immediately destroy the patient's best vision. When used in appropriate areas, it slows or stops the deterioration in all but 3 to 4 percent of the cases.

Prognosis

Several generations ago, people did not associate diabetes with blindness. The disease was so poorly controlled, patients generally died before severe damage occurred in the eyes. Today, although diabetes is not yet curable, it is better controlled. Therefore, less damage occurs to the body, but retinopathy is likely to develop. If it is detected early, diabetic retinopathy responds to treatment.

According to the American Academy of Ophthalmology, 50 percent of persons with diabetes develop some damage to the blood vessels in the retina after having had the disease for ten years. In patients who have had the disease for twenty years, the percentage goes up to 90 percent. Any retinal damage done by the disease is permanent, and there is no way to restore the lost vision.

CHAPTER 10

Glaucoma

The term "glaucoma" defines a family of diseases causing progressive damage to the optic nerve. Simply stated, glaucoma is marked by high pressure within the eyeball, but this is not true in all cases. Persons most likely to develop glaucoma are: (1) persons over age forty, (2) persons in families known to have the disease, and (3) persons who are very nearsighted.

Glaucoma destroys peripheral vision. Figure 10.1 illustrates vision loss from glaucoma. If the disease is detected early and treated, the loss of peripheral vision can be considerably less than what is shown. The illustration's black areas represent scotomas, or blind spots, perceived by the patient as the absence of sight, not as black areas.

Although glaucoma is uncommon in persons under forty, it can certainly occur at younger ages. Two percent of adults develop this disease. While there is a hereditary factor involved, children born to a parent with glaucoma do not always develop the disease. People with a parent who has glaucoma should have annual exams before the age of forty and more frequently later in life.

There are three types of glaucoma, each categorized by onset. The first is a very slow, painless, and, for the most part, undetectable development of the disease.

The second type is a sudden and painful onset. **If this happens, it is critical to get professional help within twenty-four hours, or irreparable damage may occur in one's peripheral vision.**

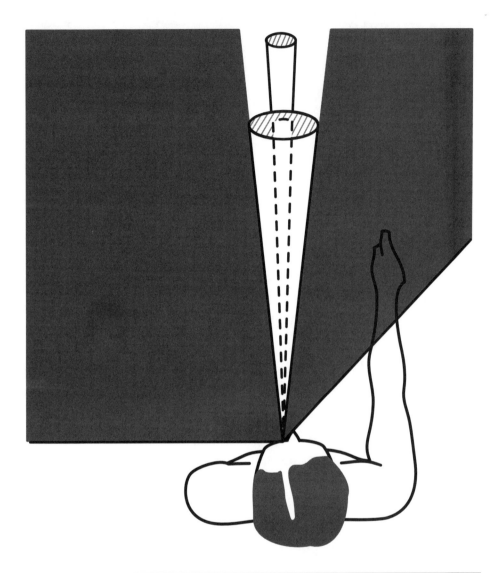

Figure 10.1: Loss of Peripheral Vision Caused by Glaucoma
Loss can be either less than or greater than what is shown.

The third type is the most common, but unfortunately few people recognize the symptoms as indicating glaucoma. Vision becomes blurred, misty, or foggy, and this may occur only intermittently. Since the problem comes and goes, people who experience these symptoms are often slow to seek help. A second symptom is pain, but it may not be sharp or even centered in the eye. The pain may be located anywhere from the forehead to the cheeks and it may be so mild as to cause no alarm. A third symptom is seeing halos, usually at night while looking at distant lights.

Important note: All three of these symptoms can come and go intermittently, causing the victim to delay getting help. These same symptoms occur with other diseases; therefore, consulting a professional immediately is very important if any one of them occurs. Hours can make the difference in arresting irreparable damage to the peripheral vision. Phone an eye doctor, describe your symptoms to the office assistant, and insist on an immediate appointment.

How Glaucoma Damages the Eye

The eyes, which are filled with fluid, produce new fluid and discharge old fluid. When production matches discharge, pressure inside the eye remains constant. Eyes have several regulatory mechanisms for maintaining uniform pressure, but when these mechanisms malfunction, the pressure can rise, causing the eyeball to expand like a balloon. The eyeball is somewhat elastic, so the change in size isn't much of a problem to the eyeball itself. By contrast, the optic nerve is inflexible. Whereas the tissue inside the optic nerve is very delicate, the covering around the optic nerve is rather tough and rigid. As the eyeball expands with an increase in pressure, the optic nerve does not expand. The result is that the eyeball begins to tear loose from the optic nerve (see Figure 10.2).

Recall from Chapter 3 that two kinds of light-sensing cells exist on the surface of the retina: rods and cones. Each rod and each

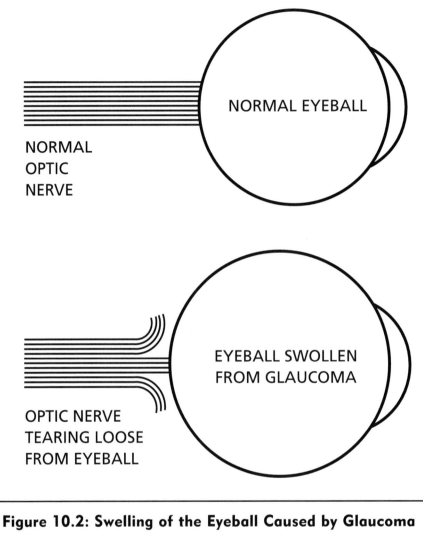

NORMAL EYEBALL

NORMAL
OPTIC
NERVE

EYEBALL SWOLLEN
FROM GLAUCOMA

OPTIC NERVE
TEARING LOOSE
FROM EYEBALL

Figure 10.2: Swelling of the Eyeball Caused by Glaucoma
The swelling causes the optic nerve to tear loose.

cone is connected to the brain through the optic nerve by tiny
nerve fibers. The arrangement of these fibers inside the optic nerve
is the same as their arrangement on the surface of the retina.
Fibers from the fovea form the center of the optic nerve. Fibers
from the macula surround those from the fovea. Fibers from the

rods, in the peripheral portion of vision, lie near the outer covering of the optic nerve.

When the optic nerve tears loose from the eyeball, its outer casing comes loose first. As pressure increases, fibers just inside the outer covering begin to break. Then fibers toward the center of the optic nerve begin to break. The last to break are the fibers from the macula and fovea, located in the very center of the optic nerve. When these fibers break, vision is destroyed. The typical patient with glaucoma loses peripheral vision first, but unless surgery or medication controls the disease, the damage can leave the patient totally blind.

Any damage done by glaucoma is permanent. Vision already lost will not be regained. Treatment can only prevent the disease from progressing.

Tests for Glaucoma

The usual test for glaucoma involves measuring the pressure in the eyeball. This test alone does not detect all types of glaucoma, for example, a low-pressure type of glaucoma. A full battery of tests for glaucoma involves visual examination of the optic nerve, or disk, for damage, and testing the field of vision for blind spots.

Treatment

Glaucoma is treatable, and many victims can live a normal life if they use medication as prescribed. Medication includes eyedrops specific for the type of glaucoma, oral medication, or both. After the patient has taken medication for months or years, the condition sometimes appears to improve. The eyeball pressure seems to stabilize. This can happen, but glaucoma can recur. On the other hand, when damage is extensive, additional deterioration may occur even after the pressure is controlled.

Sometimes surgery is the prescribed treatment. The procedure involves installing a safety valve that allows pressure to escape when the pressure becomes too high. Surgery always involves risks, and since medication controls pressure without risk, it remains the preferred treatment, as long as the pressure can be checked regularly. For this reason, a patient with glaucoma planning an extended trip to a remote part of the world might elect to take the risk of surgery before leaving.

CHAPTER 11

Macular Degeneration

The term "macular degeneration" describes a large group of related diseases that affect the macula, causing loss of central vision. Discussion in this chapter is limited to two major types: Stargardt's disease and age-related macular degeneration.

Numerous other conditions besides macular degeneration also affect the macula, thus also causing loss of central vision. A few of these are macular atrophy, macular edema, macular lesions, and cone atrophy. If the term "macula" is a part of one's visual diagnosis, he or she is among those patients who have lost some or all of their central vision. The coping techniques used by patients with macular degeneration are also applicable to those with other forms of macular disease.

Macular degeneration destroys central vision. Figure 11.1 illustrates the **maximum** loss of central vision caused by the disease. The black in the drawing illustrates the blind area, or scotoma, which the patient perceives as a loss of vision.

Stargardt's Disease

Stargardt's disease is one of the macular diseases labeled "juvenile," because its onset usually occurs during the childhood or teen years. It can occur, however, as late as age forty.

Stargardt's disease is hereditary. The hereditary pattern is autosomal recessive. This means that the disease occurs only to children whose parents are **both** carriers. Neither carrier need have the disease, but each child born to this couple will have a 25 percent chance of developing the disease. This doesn't mean that 25 percent of their children **will** develop the disease. Indeed, a couple, both of whom are carriers, can have several perfectly normal children in whom the disease never develops. On the other hand, one or all of their children **may** develop the disease.

In 1997, researchers identified the gene that causes Stargardt's. Interestingly, the research found that the same gene causes 16 percent of the age-related form of macular degeneration. This was the first "proof" that these diseases have a genetic base, although Stargardt's disease has long been known to be hereditary. Its genetic origin was apparent in its pattern of occurrence.

Stargardt's disease usually starts in the fovea of the retina and spreads outward into the macula. It can also start in the macula and spread both outward and inward. In both cases, only the macula and fovea are destroyed.

The latter way is how it developed in my eyes. For a time, I had a doughnut-shaped blind spot around the fovea. The fovea worked fine, so I had 20/20 vision for several years after the onset of the disease. But eventually, the center of the doughnut (the fovea) also deteriorated, and the disease spread outward, destroying the entire macula.

The disease affects both eyes, although it begins in one. A characteristic of the disease is that the fovea and macula turn into a gray-green mass of scar tissue containing flecks of yellow or white. These flecks are deposits of a substance called drusen, which probably consists of waste material produced by the retina's living cells. The earliest indication of onset is discoloration in the fovea and macula (the yellow spot). Discoloration of this area can occur for other reasons, so discoloration does not automatically signify macular degeneration.

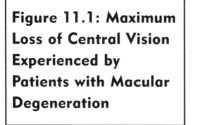

Figure 11.1: Maximum Loss of Central Vision Experienced by Patients with Macular Degeneration

Typically, Stargardt's disease is active for about ten years. The rate of deterioration and the degree of damage to the macula vary. Usually, the disease destroys tissue in the fovea and macula for ten years and then stabilizes.

My Case History

In my case, discoloration of the macula developed in late 1959, when I was thirty-one. I began experiencing vision problems in 1962. The first diagnosis of macular degeneration came in late 1965, and by this time deterioration was bilateral (both eyes). By 1968, distortion developed, caused by swelling on the surface of the retina. At this time, my best corrected visual acuity was 20/30. My visual acuity would have measured worse had the disease started in the fovea. By December 1970, my visual acuity had dropped to 20/80 and 20/60. By 1976, it had dropped to 20/120 and become stable. Ten years later, additional deterioration occurred.

When this happened, I complained to my low-vision specialist that the disease wasn't supposed to reactivate and continue its destructive work after ten years! The doctor asked, "Are you sure the disease read the same books you read?" Apparently not. My visual acuity continued to deteriorate to its present 20/240.

Although they are different diseases, Stargardt's disease and the "dry" form of age-related macular degeneration are very similar. The bright side of this problem is that neither Stargardt's disease nor age-related macular degeneration destroys peripheral vision. This, to my knowledge, holds true for all other forms of macular degeneration.

Macular Degeneration International (MDI), a support group for persons with Stargardt's and other macular diseases (see Appendix B), was organized in 1991. Sufferers of these disorders will benefit from membership in the group, which monitors research in the field and informs members of new developments. The prevalence of Stargardt's disease is unknown, but MDI estimates the number of victims in the United States at thirty thousand to fifty thousand.

In the community of the visually impaired, persons with cataracts are comparatively fortunate. Surgery will correct their vision problems. Of those remaining, the person with macular degeneration is best able to overcome the effects of the disease. There is absolutely no argument that the person who loses peripheral vision has a more severe disability than those who lose central vision. True, this gives the person with macular degeneration no comfort, but it might help to know that there are people out there who may suffer more! In fact, since Stargardt's disease usually begins during childhood, these patients must contend with their disability for a longer period.

Age-Related Macular Degeneration

Age-related macular degeneration (also called AMD or sometimes ARMD) was first named "senile macular degeneration." The word "senile" distinguished the disorder from the juvenile types, but because senior citizens today exercise more clout, doctors renamed the disease with a less offensive term. I guess they figured, why risk getting bopped on the head with a cane or a purse?

AMD appears to be caused by a substance called **drusen** that collects under the macula between the light-sensing cells and the layer of blood vessels beneath them. Drusen may be the waste product of the retinal cells in the macula. Researchers haven't yet established whether the drusen kills the cells above it or only interferes with the transfer of nutrients from the blood vessels to the light-sensing cells. In either case, the light-sensing cells in the macula die.

AMD is the leading cause of vision loss among Americans over eighteen. Diabetes remains the leading cause of vision loss in the general population since it strikes all ages, but age-related macular degeneration ranks number one among adults. The onset of AMD occurs after age fifty and, more commonly, between sixty and seventy-five.

AMD never totally blinds a person. It destroys central vision, which is the sharp vision, but leaves the peripheral vision virtually untouched. When central vision is destroyed, the patient progressively loses reading ability. He or she can still read large print during the early stages of the disease, but ultimately print even one to two inches tall will give trouble. The patient can't thread a needle or see movies or TV, and he can't pass a vision test, so he loses his driver's license. The recognition of faces — even those of close friends and relatives — becomes difficult. It is easy to understand how this disease severely disables its victim.

How Prevalent Is It?

Macular Degeneration International reports that there are at least 13 million cases of age-related macular degeneration in the United States today, with 750,000 new cases reported each year. The actual number is probably much higher, because many cases go unreported. Many senior citizens, or their loved ones, assume that the seniors' eyes are simply wearing out from age. This is untrue. Eyes do not wear out. Disease or accidents, not age, destroy vision. Age impacts vision, but only disease or accidents destroy it.

Calling the disease "age-related" seems to support the idea that the deterioration is caused by age. For this reason, I prefer the original name, "senile macular degeneration," even if it sounds derogatory (in fact, the word "senile" originally just meant "of or relating to old age"; only later did it take on the added connotation of a loss of mental faculty). Whereas both terms are associated with age, the label "age-related" seems to imply a causal relationship.

There are two types of AMD: the wet type and the dry type. In the wet type, hemorrhage of the retina occurs; in the dry type, no hemorrhage occurs. Ninety percent of cases are the dry type, and 10 percent are the wet type. At present, only the wet type is treatable. Laser treatments can control its progress if it is detected early.

Each year, doctors declare twenty-two thousand new patients legally blind from AMD. All of these patients are over sixty, and many die before extensive damage is done. Of men who live to be seventy-five, about one out of every four will develop AMD. Women are even less fortunate. Of women who reach seventy-five, about one out of every three will develop AMD. The incidence rises to 40 percent for people older than seventy-five. Obviously, with people living longer these days, the risk of losing one's vision to AMD is increasing.

Early Detection

In addition to laser treatment, certain drugs are beginning to show promise of helping people with the wet form of the disease. **So if you suspect you have developed AMD, seeing an ophthalmologist who specializes in diseases of the retina is critical. Additionally, the window of time during which laser treatment or drugs can be effective is very short. Many doctors believe it is limited to only a few days after distortion in the vision occurs.**

Fortunately, it is possible to detect the disease's onset. There are two clear signals: (1) One of the earliest is distortion of the vision, where lines or objects that are straight instead appear bent or crooked. Distortion is caused by swelling on the surface of the retina, brought about by AMD. (2) Any gradual or rapid loss of visual ability after the age of fifty. If this happens to you, have it checked out.

Self-testing methods are available. See Figure 11.2 for an example of a self-testing grid similar to what a doctor might give you. Check one eye at a time. Cover the eye without touching the eyeball or putting pressure on it. Look at the center of the grid. Do all the lines appear straight, or do some appear crooked? Then test the other eye. If you detect any crookedness in a straight line, or if some of the lines disappear, schedule an appointment with a retina specialist. Ask to be tested for macular degeneration. If you have developed the disorder, inquire whether you are a candidate for laser treatment.

How Seriously Will Vision Be Impacted?

AMD begins in one eye, but it will usually affect both. Doctors insist that some patients with a very mild form of the disease may escape loss in one eye, but I am inclined to speculate that these patients simply die before the disease affects the second eye.

AMD does not destroy peripheral vision. Since peripheral vision provides a visual acuity ranging from 20/200 to 20/2000, patients can expect their acuity to drop to about 20/200. The worst in a patient whom I tested, with one exception, was 20/240. This was the test result after the patient learned how to use eccentric viewing.

I have read dozens of ophthalmology reports indicating visual acuity test results of 20/6000 on persons with AMD. The reports said, "The patient can see hand movements at twelve inches." (This is the same as 20/6000.) These reports simply aren't true. People with AMD see better than this. If doctors were better informed about subnormal vision, they would realize the inaccuracy of a diagnosis of 20/6000.

Recall that a person is forced to use a white cane between

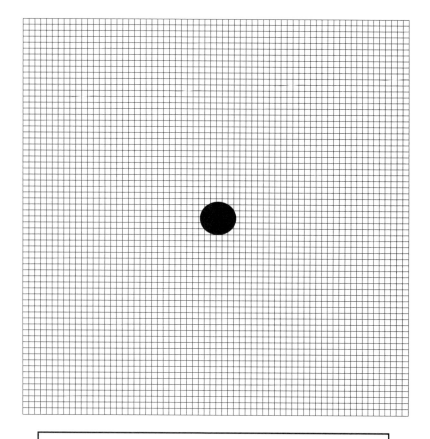

Figure 11.2: A Test Grid for Detecting the Onset of Macular Degeneration

20/800 and 20/1200. The patients with AMD whom a doctor measures at 20/6000 walked into the doctor's office without feeling their way through the door. They walked around any obstacles in their path to take a seat in the examining chair — all without help. They can't be as bad off as 20/6000! In reality, after AMD has completed its destructive work and the patient learns eccentric viewing, his visual acuity will be no worse than 20/240.

These doctors are trying to test **central** vision, when in fact AMD has destroyed it. Naturally, if the patient isn't taught eccentric viewing before his vision testing, he can't see even the chart, and certainly not the letters on it. His blind spot may be four feet in diameter at a distance of twenty feet. Some doctors tell patients with AMD to "try looking to the side." However, telling a person to look to the side of what he wants to see is not teaching him how to use his peripheral vision. "Telling" doesn't overcome the reflex to look directly at what one wants to see, nor does it overcome the habit of using the eyes in a certain way for sixty or seventy years.

Doctors occasionally report seeing AMD that has spread outward beyond the macula. Such an occurrence is rare. I have seen only one such case in twenty years. Patients with the wet form of AMD are more likely to experience this excessive deterioration. Even in these unusual cases, the disease does not destroy the entire retina.

Research: Is Help on the Way?

Earlier I mentioned laser surgery as a treatment for those who develop wet-type AMD. Laser therapy proved to be of great benefit, but high-intensity laser killed light-sensing cells wherever it was used. This limited its use to areas on the retina away from the fovea. In April 2000 the FDA approved a new laser treatment for the wet form of AMD. It is called visudyne therapy. A laser-activated drug called verteporfin is injected into the bloodstream. The drug adheres to the inside wall of leaking blood vessels. After a few minutes, a low-energy laser is directed into the eye. The laser activates the drug to close the blood vessels. The treatment can be used on 40 to 60 percent of persons with the wet form of AMD. This low-intensity laser does not kill retinal cells.

Research is ongoing about the possibilities of using other drugs — for example, interferon and thalidomide — to stop the growth of these extraneous blood vessels in the wet form of AMD.

Interferon is used in the treatment of cancer. Thalidomide, originally developed as a sedative and hypnotic drug, is the drug that caused thousands of birth defects during the 1950s and 1960s. For this reason, any woman in her childbearing years is required to maintain use of a dependable contraceptive method if she is treated with thalidomide for any condition. In addition, radiation administered in low doses over a period of several days is under study as a means of preventing growth of the extraneous retinal blood vessels that are the culprit in wet-type AMD.

For those with dry-type macular degeneration, several developments promise help in the near to distant future. Note: It is unlikely there will ever be any kind of treatment for patients who have had this disease for more than a year, but talk to your doctor about the following treatments. As far as I know, all the treatments listed below apply to both wet and dry AMD.

1. A promising new treatment for both the wet and dry forms of AMD went into clinical trials during 1999. Doctors noticed that after laser surgery for the wet form, the drusen beneath the macula disappeared. A high-intensity laser is used in this surgery, and while it stops the hemorrhage of the wet form, it also kills light-sensing cells. Doctors speculate that the heat generated by the laser causes the drusen to disappear. The procedure under clinical study involves using a low-intensity laser that generates enough heat to remove the drusen but does not destroy light-sensing cells. This appears to be the most promising treatment developed thus far. Test results should be available soon.

2. The retina, along with the male prostate, contains more zinc than any other tissue in the body. There are some indications that taking zinc may help to slow the disease, but

excessive doses of zinc can be dangerous. Take zinc only under the direction of a doctor.

3. Researchers have injected healthy retinal cells into the eyes of rats whose retinas have been destroyed, and the cells have "taken root" and functioned. The technique is now being tested on humans. The latest reports from this research indicate that the injected cells "take root," but the cells do not connect to the brain through the optic nerve. Research continues in this area.

4. Researchers report that surgical removal of scar tissue beneath the retina and of a layer of light-sensing cells on the surface of the retina has resulted in the regeneration of functioning cells. The technique looks promising, but it is still strictly experimental.

5. The fall 1995 issue of <u>Fighting Blindness News</u> (published by the RP [Retinitis Pigmentosa] Foundation Fighting Blindness) announced research findings indicating that eating dark-green leafy vegetables like spinach, collard greens, kale, and mustard greens may reduce the risk of developing AMD. Research indicated that people who ate only two or three half-cup servings per week significantly reduced their risk of developing AMD. Those who ate five or six servings per week reduced their risk factor by 50 percent. Those who took antioxidants in pill form instead of "eating their spinach" did not attain these results.

   Since taking antioxidants in pill form did not help, researchers do not know if these results were caused by the antioxidants in dark-green leafy vegetables or by some other substance they contain. If it is the antioxidants that are the helpful ingredient, then researchers report that a cup of black or green tea contains the same amount of antioxidants as a half cup of spinach. Not all tea is black or green. Check the label before you buy.

Note that eating dark-green leafy vegetables is not promoted as a **cure,** but as a **preventive** for those who have not yet developed the disease.

6. The back of the eye contains layers. The inside layer is made up of light-sensing cells. The next layer is a mass of blood vessels. AMD develops when this blood-vessel layer deteriorates and destroys the light-sensing cells above it. Since it is only one layer that deteriorates — the blood-vessel layer beneath the macula — doctors have tried a procedure that detaches the retina and moves the macula over so that it has sound blood-vessel tissue beneath it. When the surgery is done early, just as deterioration is beginning, the macula is saved. The newly located light-sensing cells over the bad tissue at the macula's previous location will die, but the sharper vision provided by the fovea and macula are preserved. This research is still in the experimental stage and is not yet ready for general application.

To keep up with new research, consider joining a support group related to macular diseases. Two are listed in Appendix B: the Association for Macular Diseases and a newer organization, Macular Degeneration International. Additionally, one of the very best sources of information about research is the newsletter published by the RP Foundation Fighting Blindness also listed in Appendix B.

CHAPTER 12

Retinitis Pigmentosa[2]

The term "retinitis pigmentosa," usually shortened to RP, defines a group of hereditary retinal diseases that destroy light-sensing cells on the retina. The most common symptoms of RP result from the destruction of rods in the peripheral area of the patient's vision. Rods provide night vision and peripheral vision, so when these cells cease to function, night blindness and tunnel vision develop. Figure 12.1 shows the **progressive** loss of peripheral vision caused by RP. The black areas in the drawings indicate blind spots, perceived by the patient as the absence of sight, not as black spots.

Another form of retinitis pigmentosa predominantly affects the cones first. When this happens, symptoms occur very similar to those associated with macular degeneration; that is, central vision is lost first. This type, called "macular retinitis pigmentosa," is not the same disease as macular degeneration, but its impact on one's vision is the same. Therefore, the patient with macular retinitis pigmentosa needs to follow the recommendations for coping with macular degeneration, instead of the ones for retinitis pigmentosa. Readers should consult with a doctor about the specifics of their disease to select the treatment and coping options that will work best for them.

A common feature of RP is a gradual loss of light-sensing cells. If predominately rod damage occurs first, a loss of visual acuity can also occur before field loss is complete.

Normally, it takes years for the disease to cause serious loss of sight. Most individuals with RP lose vision gradually over a period

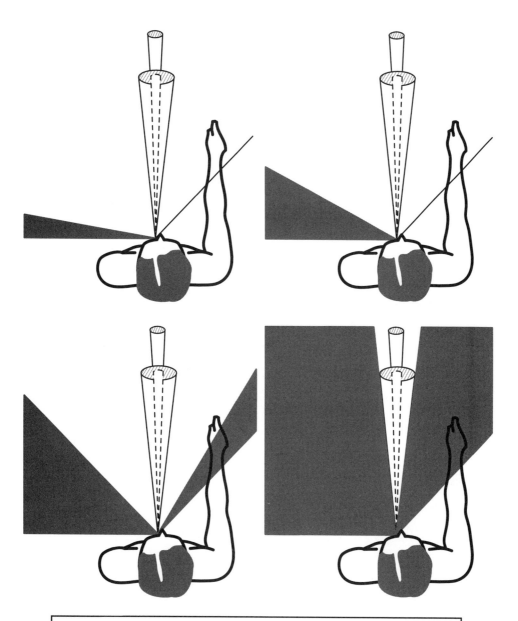

Figure 12.1: Progressive Loss of Peripheral Vision Caused by Retinitis Pigmentosa

In advanced cases, the loss can be greater than what is illustrated.

of years or even decades. Often, vision loss occurs so slowly that one cannot determine additional loss from one annual exam to the next. The rate of deterioration is often — but not always — about the same within a given family.

It is not unusual for people with RP to develop cataracts. The reason for this is not clearly understood. (See Chapter 8, "Cataracts.")

What Causes RP?

Researchers believe that RP is caused by mutations of certain genes required for vision. They have identified several RP gene mutations. They believe these gene mutations send faulty signals to the retinal cells and cause them to deteriorate. Identification of these mutations opens the door to other breakthroughs in treatment and prevention.

How Is RP Inherited?

RP is hereditary. Sometimes RP occurs in a family where the tendency is unknown to have existed. Very recently, researchers have found two genes located on different chromosomes (chromosome numbers eleven and six) that cause cases to occur in families without a history of the disease. This is the first time research has shown that a disease can be caused by different genes located on different chromosomes.

RP can be inherited in four different ways: autosomal dominant inheritance; autosomal recessive inheritance; X-linked inheritance (normally called sex-linked); and the newly discovered digenic type, inherited from unaffected parents. Each type of inheritance causes a different pattern of affected family members. For example, unaffected parents could have affected children. Affected parents could have both affected and unaffected children. In some families, only males will develop the disease, but females will carry the trait, even though they do not develop the disease. All children affected by the disease will not be affected the same way. One may show mild symptoms, while another shows severe ones. A child can have a mild form and not be aware of it. Any time RP occurs in a family, all members of the family are at risk.

The RP Foundation Fighting Blindness provides special literature on the subject of heredity. It also supplies the names of doctors who offer genetic counseling. You can find the organization's address in Appendix B.

How Prevalent Is It?

The RP Foundation Fighting Blindness estimates that one hundred thousand cases of RP exist in the United States today. In the family of diseases labeled "RP," subtypes are known to exist that affect only a hundred people, while another type may affect a thousand. As with so many other diseases, there are people who have it but remain unaware that they do.

Does Treatment Exist?

Presently, no cure exists for RP. A six-year clinical study of RP reported in June 1993 that taking a specified daily vitamin A supplement (in the form of vitamin A palmitate) slowed the decline of vision in persons with RP. The treatment does not cure the disease, nor can significant decreases in the disease's progress be seen between annual exams, but it does slow the disease.

The November 1999 <u>Update</u> of the <u>Fighting Blindness Newsletter</u> reported the safety results of a long-term study of the vitamin A treatment. It concluded that for persons aged eighteen to fifty-four (the age group studied), taking up to twenty-five thousand IU (international units) of vitamin A per day was safe for twelve years (the period of time studied). However, be advised that no one should undertake this treatment without first consulting a doctor. Blood levels of vitamin A must be closely monitored, and the liver must be checked annually for damage.

Doctors once thought that protecting the eyes from light slowed the disease. Most doctors no longer support this theory, except possibly in cases of extremely intense sunlight, such as that found over snow or on beaches.

How Seriously Will Vision Be Impacted?

RP can lead to blindness, if blindness is defined as a total loss of sight. Many people with RP lose all light perception in their later years, but many do not. My friend Ira Bossert, who operates the low-vision-aid supplier Bossert Specialties (see Appendix B), is a good example. I met Ira in 1979. He had tunnel vision then, but he still enjoyed travel and object vision. By 1986, most of his vision was gone. Today, Ira is in his sixties. His travel vision is gone, but he still enjoys enough vision to use video visual aids for print and large-print displays on a computer.

Coping with RP

Anyone with RP should do what he or she can to remain in good general health and avoid excessive use of drugs of any kind.

Persons with RP should consult their own physician, who knows their case personally. Those who experience the loss of peripheral vision would do well to work with an orientation and mobility instructor to learn adaptive skills. The state commission for the blind, sometimes called visual services, can help locate an orientation and mobility instructor.

Having night blindness does not automatically mean a person has RP, though night blindness is a common symptom of the disease. Night blindness means more than simply being blind at night. It also relates to the inability to see in diminished light, as in restaurants. Many patients with RP become indignant about the low-light atmosphere in restaurants. They can't see their plates or anything else! Persons with night blindness need not feel restricted from the pleasures of dining out in low-light atmospheres. See Chapter 16, "Light," for a discussion of battery-operated lighted magnifiers suitable for reading menus in dark restaurants.

If you don't require magnification, but do need more light than many restaurants provide, other options exist. Gone are the days when the only portable lights available were bulky flashlights and propane lanterns. Dozens of small, battery-operated, inconspicuous, surprisingly bright lights exist on the market for camping and reading. Some of these might be appropriate to take along to a restaurant to use for reading the menu or seeing your plate. Some can be set on the table in front of you; others are handheld. Lanterns that contain L.E.D. bulbs are the best. L.E.D. bulbs offer an ambient, pure-white light, and the batteries last up to twice as long as with incandescent lights. You will probably want to make sure the light provided by any such product aims down — directly at your plate or menu — rather than lighting up the whole room!

To discuss options for portable lighting, contact any reputable outdoor-equipment retailer. A good one is REI, which has locations in most cities. You can also visit their Web site: www.rei.com. For other styles of portable lights, contact a good bookstore. The larger ones offer lights designed for reading while traveling.

If shopping for a portable light doesn't yield exactly the product you desire, consider making one of your own! See Appendix C for instructions on building a battery-operated "plate light," so-called because it lights up only your plate in a dark restaurant — not the entire room!

Part IV

Coping Techniques and Equipment

Each of the chapters in this section introduces a coping technique or piece of equipment for persons with low vision. At the beginning of most chapters, a chart is included to rate that technique's or item's appropriateness for helping with a given disease. The chart presents a scale from 1 to 10. A rating of 1 means "little if any help for someone with this disease." A rating of 10 means "very effective for someone with this disease." A rating of 4–5–6, therefore, means "moderately helpful for someone with this disease." Other ratings can be gauged accordingly.

The last column on the chart refers to special notes located below the chart. The notes qualify or add additional information. Read the notes that apply to you.

CHAPTER 13

The First Principle: Get Closer

Disease	Usefulness (scale 1–10)	See note number
Cataracts	10	1
Diabetic retinopathy	10	1
Glaucoma	10	1
Macular degeneration	10	1
Retinitis pigmentosa	10	1

Scale

1 =   Offers little if any help for someone with this disease.

4–5–6 = Moderately effective for someone with this disease.

10 =   Very effective for someone with this disease.

(Other ratings can be gauged accordingly.)

Note

1. With one exception, getting closer is helpful to everyone, even the normally sighted. It is a principle of vision. The exception is the person who has lost most of his or her peripheral vision, leaving only a very narrow field of tunnel vision. In this case, getting closer doesn't help. Usually, doing so will handicap the person even more. If one's field of vision is so restricted that standing six feet away she sees

only a person's face, she may see only the nose if she moves up to three feet.

The First Principle

The first principle in dealing with vision loss is to **get closer.** Recall the information in Chapter 1 on visual acuity notation. The person who sees a 200-size letter on the test chart at a distance of 20 feet can read the 100-size letter when he moves up to 10 feet. If he moves up to 2 feet, he can read the 20-size letters — the same letters a person with normal vision can read from a distance of 20 feet.

Simply put, the rule is: **Cutting the distance in half doubles what a person can see.** This principle is tremendously important to understand and use. Let's consider a person who wants to watch TV. Normally he sits 10 feet from the set. If he moves to 5 feet from the set, he can see the screen twice as well. If he moves up to $2\frac{1}{2}$ feet (30 inches) from the set, he can see it 4 times as well as he did from 10 feet. If he moves up to 15 inches, once again he doubles what he can see. This is called "approach magnification," and the principle holds true no matter what the distance. As an object comes closer to the eye, it seems to get larger. The brain knows the object isn't getting larger, but the eye doesn't know this. As far as the eye is concerned, the object grows enormous when it comes very close.

Theoretically, someone who is a true 20/200 needs 10-power magnification to see as well as someone with normal vision. (This principle will be discussed in detail later.) Consider the task of viewing a friend across the room. From 20 feet, a person who is partially sighted can see her friend, but she may not be able to recognize him. However, if she moves up to 1¾ inches from the target person, she sees him 128 times better than she did from 20 feet. This is 128-power magnification, and a person with a visual acuity of 20/200 needs magnification of only 10-power to see as well as the normally sighted.

Of course, people don't typically get this close to others they're trying to recognize. The above example simply serves to illustrate the effectiveness of this technique. Even if you move to within 7½ inches from someone, you've increased the magnification 32 times from what you could see at 20 feet. Approach magnification helps everyone (except the person with serious field loss). So remember, if your visual acuity is 20/200, standing 2 feet from something allows you to see it exactly as a person with normal vision would see it from 20 feet.

What Else Should I Know?

Overcoming the consequences of vision loss often means nothing more than getting off one's duff and moving closer! Want to see someone's face? Get closer. Want to see if something is clean? Get closer. Can't see what is being written? Get closer. Every time you move closer, you see better.

To be realistic, other variables are at work in getting closer. When one moves very near the target object, his eyes may not focus at that distance. He may see the object better, but still not sharply. However, people can live their lives and do many activities without seeing things sharply. The visually impaired need to accept the fact that they will never see things sharply again — and then use the technique of getting closer to maximize what they **can** see and do. A woman in Austin once complained that she could no longer see her husband. She was surprised when I asked her if her husband still kissed her. When she answered yes, I suggested she open her eyes! Getting that close solves most vision problems.

The value of getting closer increases when it is used with other coping techniques and equipment (more will be said later about combining coping techniques).

Persons who have lost central vision must use eccentric viewing in combination with this technique.

Never discount the value of getting closer, one of the simplest and easiest techniques to use.

CHAPTER 14

Eccentric Viewing[3]

Disease	Usefulness (scale 1–10)	See note number
Cataracts	4–5–6	1
Diabetic retinopathy	4–5–6	2
Glaucoma	1	3
Macular degeneration	10	4
Retinitis pigmentosa	1	3

Scale

1 = Offers little if any help for someone with this disease.

4–5–6 = Moderately effective for someone with this disease.

10 = Very effective for someone with this disease.

(Other ratings can be gauged accordingly.)

Notes

1. Sometimes cataracts are denser in one part of the lens than in other parts. When this is true, eccentric viewing may be of help.

2. Diabetic retinopathy is always more destructive to one part of the retina. As the disease progresses, the area of the retina that provides more functional vision may change, but some part of the retina will work better than others. Eccentric viewing for most of these persons is effective.

3. Generally, persons who lose peripheral vision are not helped by this technique, but exceptions do exist. Even if most object vision is gone in the peripheral fields, there may still be functioning retinal tissue that can be used, for example, to read with a video visual aid. These patients should give the technique a chance. While it may prove useless for independent travel, they may enjoy enough functional vision in the peripheral fields to perform other tasks.

4. For persons with macular disease, eccentric viewing is the most important coping technique. They must master it! It is the key to their success or failure in overcoming the effects of the disease.

What Is Eccentric Viewing?

Eccentric viewing is not looking directly at what one wants to see. Expressed another way, eccentric viewing is looking at things with one's peripheral vision. It is used to compensate for the loss of central vision.

Of all the techniques one needs to overcome macular degeneration, none is higher on the list than eccentric viewing. **Persons with macular degeneration should use eccentric viewing in conjunction with all other coping techniques.** As shown in the chart above, the technique also proves useful to certain persons with other diseases.

Chapter 11 discussed how macular degeneration kills cells on the retina. The cells in the macula and fovea die, so the patient is left with a totally blind spot. Diabetic retinopathy also destroys this part of the retina. Retinitis pigmentosa and glaucoma destroy peripheral vision, but these diseases can also damage central vision before one's peripheral fields are severely restricted.

Recall that the fovea, located in the center of the macula, provides the only 20/20 vision in a normal eye. It provides the only truly sharp vision in the eye's 180-degree field of view. Because this is true, people develop the habit of turning their eyes to look directly at what they want to see. If someone with a healthy eye wants to see a person's face, she fixates on the face. In other words, the eyes move until they point directly at the face, thereby focusing light onto the fovea. The person with macular degeneration has lost or is losing this part of the retina. The fovea and macula are dead or dying. When these persons look directly at a target object, such as a person's face, they see nothing. Light entering the eye is being focused on dead tissue. (During the early stages of macular degeneration, a person's face or another target object may only partially disappear or become blurred.)

How to Use Eccentric Viewing

By contrast, someone using eccentric viewing doesn't look directly at a person's face. Instead, he looks at the person's shoulder or off to the side of the face. This puts the blind spot at shoulder level or off to the side, so he sees the face in his peripheral vision. To do this, move the eyes only enough so that light reflected from the face is focused onto the retinal tissue **beside** the macula, but **not directly on it.** See Figure 14.1.

There is a trick to using eccentric viewing. When people are told to look to the left or right side of what they want to see, invariably they turn their heads in that direction. **Don't turn your head!** Turning the head to move the blind spot out of the way is self-defeating. The eyes simply rotate in their sockets and remain fixed on that person's face. **Never move the head! Move only the eyes!**

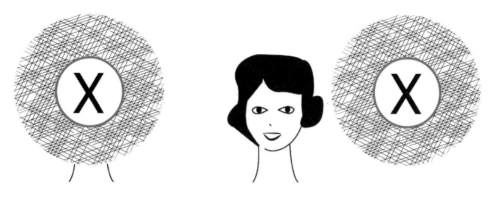

INCORRECT   CORRECT

Figure 14.1: Using Eccentric Viewing to See Faces
The "X" shows the point of fixation. The dark area shows
the position and size of the blind spot when viewing targets
six feet away after the macula is completely destroyed.

There is one direction in which a person with macular degeneration can point his eyes where he will see best. Some persons see
best when they look high and to the right. Some see best when
they look low and to the left. Others see best when they look
straight right or left. Each person must find for himself or herself
which way to point the eyes to see best. The person who turns her
head and eyes at the same time while searching for this spot of
better vision will occasionally see things better. However, if she
uses both eye and head movement, she cannot identify which way
to point her eyes to see best. If she holds her head still and moves
only her eyes, then only one variable is involved, and she quickly
learns exactly which way to point her eyes.

The following exercise will help identify exactly which way to
point your eyes to see best. Stand six feet in front of a large picture

hanging on the wall. Make sure there is plenty of light on the picture. Look at the center of the picture. A person with macular problems will see little, if anything. Now, moving the eyes only, look at the frame on the right side of the picture. Keep the eyes pointed at the frame, but **concentrate on what is seen off to the side, in the center of the picture.** Now point the eyes to the left side of the frame. Is the center of the picture any clearer? Next, look at the top of the frame, and then at the bottom. Go back and try various positions between right and left, and top and bottom. Somewhere there is a point — which only you can locate — where you can see best. Figure 14.2 illustrates how to locate this spot.

"Looking to the side" of what one wants to see is sometimes difficult for people to understand. Some people are helped by the following. If you want to see someone's face, or a teed-up golf ball, recall the direction the eyes should point to see best. Imagine there is a black "X" at that spot, then look directly at the imaginary "X."

Learning eccentric viewing can be challenging, because the natural function of peripheral vision is to tell the eyes which way to move to focus light directly onto the fovea. Learning eccentric viewing means circumventing this natural reflex of the eye. But consider the rewards of mastering this challenge. Take the person who has macular problems and has lost her object vision in central fields. She has learned that she can see best when she looks high and to the right of the target object. She looks at a doorknob about ten feet away. It disappears or becomes more blurred as she looks directly at it. When this happens, she remembers to lock her head and neck in place as if in a vise. She points her nose in the direction of the target and then turns only her eyes to look at a spot on the wall three feet high and to the right of the doorknob. The doorknob comes back into view. It is not as

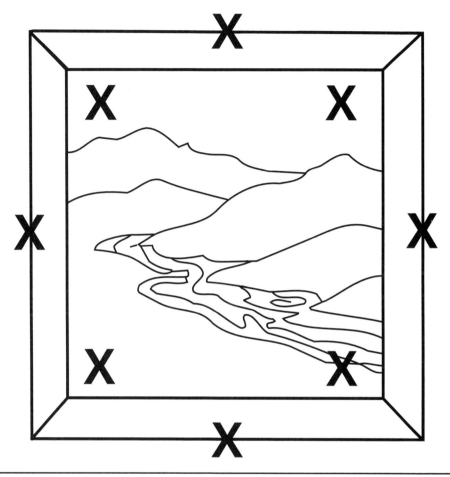

Figure 14.2: Determining Where to Point the Eyes to See Best
The "Xs" are experimental fixation points used to locate what direction one should point the eyes to see best.

sharp as it once was, but it is visible. The patient has restored her object vision simply by using her eyes in a new way!

Now consider how important mastering this technique is. Think about the task of walking downstairs. A person with macular problems looks directly at the step where he is about to put his foot. A ball is sitting there, but he doesn't see it because he is looking directly at it. Light reflected from the ball is being focused onto the dead macula. If this person instead focused his eyes on the third step away, his blind spot would fall on the third step, so the ball on the first step would be visible in his peripheral vision. He would avoid a misstep and a potentially serious accident.

Why does eccentric viewing work? Recall that visual acuity is best closer to the fovea, and gets progressively worse moving out through the macula toward the peripheral fields. Deterioration of the macula (or of other areas on the retina) is seldom uniform. The destruction doesn't start with a pinpoint and grow outward evenly in all directions, but rather leaves a blind spot that is irregularly shaped. See Figure 14.3.

When a patient turns the eyes so that light is focused on a functional part of the retina **nearer** the fovea, he or she sees better. If the eye is turned so that light is focused onto point A in Figure 14.3, the patient will see better than if light is focused on point B, and much better than if light is focused on point C.

Once you understand the principle of eccentric viewing, put it into practice. Begin practicing eccentric viewing while sitting down. When you've mastered that, practice it while walking through the house. People often ask me, "Should I practice eccentric viewing fifteen minutes every day?" The answer is no. Use it eighteen hours every day. The real challenge lies not so much in learning to do it, but rather in remembering to use it all the time. Unfortunately, eccentric viewing never becomes automatic. While learning the technique, one has to force the eyes to look away from a given target. Twenty years later, one must still use conscious effort to force the eyes off target.

Simply stated, how well the patient with macular problems learns eccentric viewing determines how disabling the disease will be in his or her life. If you learn eccentric viewing well and use it

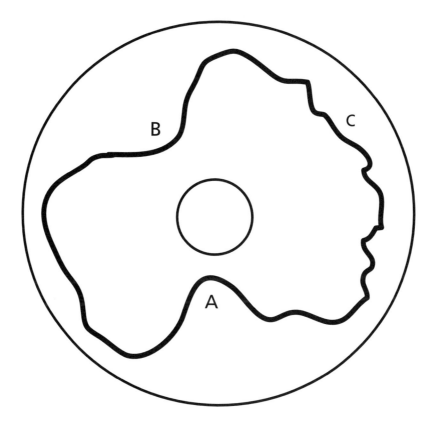

Figure 14.3: The Shape of the Blind Spot on the Macula
While this drawing shows a typical blind spot on the retina of a patient with macular degeneration, the same principle applies to diseases that destroy other parts of the retina. If a functional patch of retinal tissue can be found closer to the fovea, one's functional ability increases.

with other techniques discussed in this book, such as getting closer, then the disease will be no more than a nuisance.

People have said to me, "I have tried eccentric viewing, but it doesn't help much." Considered from one perspective, this can be true. Objects do not appear as sharp as they would if the fovea were being used. However, without eccentric viewing, the patient has a totally blind spot around the point of fixation. He or she sees nothing with that part of the retina. He doesn't even have object vision.

Here's the point: **Eccentric viewing is used to restore object vision, and other techniques or aids are used to restore sharper definition.** Get closer and use eccentric viewing, or use eccentric viewing with a telescope or magnifier. It is almost a law of subnormal vision that using one coping technique or aid by itself rarely produces dramatic results. A combination of techniques and aids offers the best results.

CHAPTER 15

Scanning

Disease	Usefulness (scale 1–10)	See note number
Cataracts	6–7–8	1
Diabetic retinopathy	8–9–10	1
Glaucoma	10	1
Macular degeneration	6–7–8	2
Retinitis pigmentosa	10	1

Scale

1 =   Offers little if any help for someone with this disease.

4–5–6 = Moderately effective for someone with this disease.

10 =   Very effective for someone with this disease.

(Other ratings can be gauged accordingly.)

Notes

1. Diabetic retinopathy and other diseases often destroy retinal tissue in a patchy manner, so that blind spots mixed with areas of better vision are common. Scanning is of value in these cases.

2. Eccentric viewing is the more valuable technique for this group, but even using eccentric viewing leaves a blind spot at the point of fixation. Scanning helps these patients to see the areas blotted out by the blind spot.

What Is Scanning?

Scanning is the basic survival tool for those who have lost peripheral vision, just as eccentric viewing is the basic survival skill for those with macular disease. Scanning is the practice of keeping the eyes continuously moving, never allowing them to remain fixed on one location. During scanning, the eyes are constantly moving from left to right or up and down.

The person who loses peripheral vision is like someone with normal vision who enters a very dark room with a flashlight. He sees only the relatively small area illuminated by the beam. Everything else remains in darkness. If he points the light at a distant wall and tries to walk across the room, he will bump his shins. The way he avoids this is to sweep the flashlight beam from his feet to eye level, illuminating items on the floor that might trip him. Likewise, he moves the light from left to right to detect obstructions that may extend into his path from the sides.

The more peripheral vision a person has lost, the more essential it is for him to master scanning. He must use his eyes as the person with normal vision would use a flashlight in a dark room. The eyes must constantly move, covering all four areas in the direction of travel. He must see what lies at his feet, what is head high, what is on his right, and what is on his left. To miss seeing objects in any one of those directions might mean bumped shins, bruised arms and shoulders, or a broken skull!

My macular degeneration requires that I look to the right of what I want to see. Over time, I discovered that I had developed the bad habit of locking my eyes onto the lane of traffic to my right so I could better see the lane straight ahead. One day in Dallas, when entering Loop 635, I was using eccentric viewing to watch the lane ahead. The lane was clear, but my blind spot, fixed to the right of my path, blocked out a car parked on the shoulder. When I finally saw the parked car, I was on top of it. There was no danger since my lane was clear. Nonetheless, when that car suddenly appeared from nowhere immediately to my right, it scared the wits out of me. I already knew that I needed to use eccentric viewing, but I learned in dramatic fashion that I needed to "cover" that blind spot by constantly moving my eyes from right to left. Any person with a blind spot somewhere in his field of view would be wise to develop the habit of scanning.

Since that event in Dallas, I have learned to use scanning. While driving down the street, doing all the things a visually impaired person must do when driving with telescopic glasses, I scan with my eyes when I am not using the scope (more explanation about the special techniques and equipment used for driving appears in later chapters). I deliberately look at the curb on the left half a block ahead. I then move my eyes back to look at the curb up ahead on the right. My eyes never stop moving. This prevents the blind spot from blotting out something, like a child, that I must see.

The person with a loss of peripheral vision who really needs this technique probably uses a white cane. While walking down a sidewalk, the cane is swung from one side of the walk to the other. Develop the skill and the rhythm of moving the eyes to either follow the cane or to move in the other direction. Every step means moving the eyes to a different location.

Persons with loss of central vision from macular problems can employ the same technique to avoid stepping on children's toys or other objects lying on the floor.

CHAPTER 16

Light

Disease	Usefulness (scale 1–10)	See note number
Cataracts	10	1
Diabetic retinopathy	10	1
Glaucoma	10	1
Macular degeneration	10	1
Retinitis pigmentosa	10	1

Scale

1 =   Offers little if any help for someone with this disease.

4–5–6 = Moderately effective for someone with this disease.

10 =   Very effective for someone with this disease.

(Other ratings can be gauged accordingly.)

Note

1. Everyone with vision loss is helped by the proper use of light, but many will be photophobic or light-sensitive. This chapter addresses both issues.

Managing Light

Light is always a problem for the visually impaired. There is either too little or too much. Either way, one must learn to manage light.

My experience indicates that persons with macular degeneration need three times more light than persons with normal vision. The same applies for any disease that has damaged the fovea and macula.

Unfortunately, many of the visually impaired are also light sensitive. This chapter describes how to cope with these matters.

Getting More Light

Add more light by using desk lamps wherever light is needed. For example, I keep a desk lamp on top of my filing cabinet so I can read file labels more easily. The labels are large print, but I still require more light. Another lamp sits beside my computer printer, and a floor lamp sits beside the chair I use while proofreading manuscripts.

Most desk lamps use sixty- to one-hundred-watt bulbs, but "student lamps," designed for two-hundred-watt bulbs, are available. These provide twice as much light, but they can also produce glare. I have one on my desk. It adequately illuminates material on the desk, but it also creates problems with glare. A piece of cardboard fastened to the lampshade protects my eyes from the strong light.

When buying lamps, avoid the small, so-called "high-intensity lights." These little lamps with metal shades get so hot they can cause blisters if touched. Lamps that have a "gooseneck" or are adjustable with "bullet shades" are best. One of these with a hundred-watt light bulb is better than a hot, high-intensity lamp. Floor lamps that provide up to three hundred watts of light are common.

Those who spend time in the kitchen should consider mounting fluorescent lights under their kitchen cabinets to light up the countertops.

Light works much like vision. The closer the light source, the more light it offers. When I needed more light on my desk, I had the overhead fluorescent fixture lowered on chains, bringing it closer to the desk. This solution worked beautifully.

Some light bulbs have a reflector built inside. Reflector bulbs come in wattages of thirty and higher. Since these bulbs concentrate all their light in one direction, they provide up to three times more light than their rating, but produce only the heat related to their wattage. In other words, a 60-watt reflector bulb will produce the equivalent of 180 watts of light, while only getting as hot as a 60-watt bulb.

Light Sensitivity

Recall from Chapter 2 how the iris works to control the amount of light entering the eye. As we age, the iris loses its ability to open and close. If it locks in wider than needed in normal light, the person will be light-sensitive, or photophobic. If locked in with a diameter too small for dim light, the person will have difficulty seeing in a dark room.

Patients who are light-sensitive should secure a pair of NOIR sunglasses (short for "NO InfraRed light"). A doctor can order them from the New York Lighthouse for the Blind, Optical Aids Service (find the address in Appendix B), but individuals who place orders must submit a prescription with the order. They retail for about $13. NOIR sunglasses are also available without a prescription from Bossert Specialties for about $24 (find the address in Appendix B).

Specifications for commonly used models are as follows:

Model 701: Can be worn over ordinary spectacles; will fit ordinary to large adult heads.

Model 101: Can be worn over ordinary spectacles; will fit average to smaller adult heads.

Model 201: Will not fit over spectacles; for teenagers and small heads.

The numbers 100, 200, and 700 define frame styles. The last two digits define color and light-filtering capability. All models filter out ultraviolet and infrared light. The 01 and 07 models have amber, contrast-enhancing lenses (the next chapter discusses contrast enhancement in detail). The number 01 designates a medium shade of amber that stops 90 percent of visible light. This is ideal for persons with macular degeneration. The number 07 designates a dark-amber color that stops 98 percent of visible light. Only extremely light-sensitive persons need glasses this dark. The number 08, dark gray, stops 99 percent of visible light. Patients with diabetic retinopathy can wear the 08 lenses, but most other patients will find them too dark. The 07 and 08 models are much more expensive than the 01 models.

NOIR glasses have wide side panels made from the same material as the lenses. If they scratch and break, return them to the dealer or to the manufacturer, Recreational Innovation, for a free replacement (find the address in Appendix B).

Using Light Properly

Figure 16.1 is a drawing of a person reading a book with a hand magnifier. It illustrates how one must learn to use light. There are specific steps to follow.

Step One: Look around and locate the primary light source. The primary source will be where most of the light is coming from. It may be a lamp, or it may be a window.

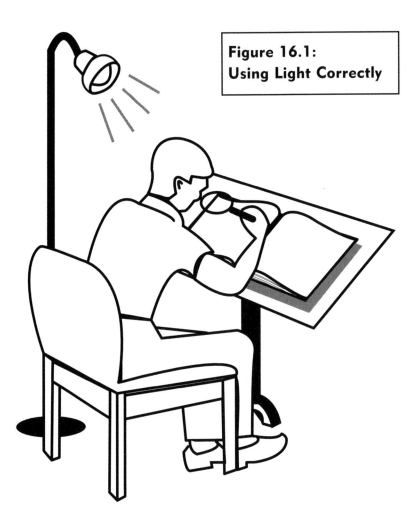

**Figure 16.1:
Using Light Correctly**

Step Two: Hold the book so that light from the primary light source falls directly on the reading material. Make sure there are no shadows on the page.

Step Three: Hold the magnifier in the hand on the opposite side of the book from the light source. In this case, the magnifier is in the right hand because the light is on the left. If the magnifier were held in the left hand, the hand and magnifier would cast a shadow on the reading material. If you favor holding the magnifier in the other hand, simply turn 180 degrees, putting the light on the other side of the book.

When magnifying spectacles are used, the principle is the same. Make sure light falls directly on the book and no shadows from your head or hands fall across the material to be read.

Reading Menus in Dark Restaurants

A lighted magnifier solves the problem of reading menus in dark restaurants. The Pike Flash-O-Lens is one of the best. A lens attached to a flashlight, it comes in +20 D. (8X) and +28 D. (11X) models. (The manufacturer refers to the magnification power offered by these models as 5X and 7X, but 8X and 11X are more accurate; see Chapter 20 for further discussion of diopters and magnification power.) This magnifier uses two D batteries. It is a "stand" magnifier, meaning that its base must stand or sit directly on the page. Hold the menu and magnifier five to eight inches from the eye. The Flash-O-Lens is available with a doctor's prescription from the New York Lighthouse for the Blind for about $45. It is also available without a prescription from Bossert Specialties for about $85. Find these addresses in Appendix B.

The same magnifier comes in 110-volt models that plug into a wall outlet. They weigh less since no batteries are required, but they are not portable because a wall outlet may not be conveniently located.

Many lighted magnifiers exist on the market today. They vary in quality and power, so make sure to get the right power for your needs. Also make sure the company offers return privileges in case the product proves unsatisfactory.

CHAPTER 17

Contrast Enhancement

Disease	Usefulness (scale 1–10)	See note number
Cataracts	10	1
Diabetic retinopathy	10	1
Glaucoma	10	1
Macular degeneration	10	1
Retinitis pigmentosa	10	1

Scale

1 = Offers little if any help for someone with this disease.

4–5–6 = Moderately effective for someone with this disease.

10 = Very effective for someone with this disease.

(Other ratings can be gauged accordingly.)

Note

1. Contrast enhancement helps everyone. It is a basic principle of vision.

Ways to Enhance Contrast

Any yellow, amber, or reddish-amber lens will improve visual ability because these colors enhance contrast. That is, they darken dark colors seen through them, but they do not darken light colors.

When dark colors get darker and light colors stay light, people see things better. Curbs and steps stand out more clearly. A dark tie will stand out more prominently against a white shirt. The light-colored pattern in a dress fabric will show up better against its dark background.

The way to enhance contrast is to wear special lenses. If you want to go first class, ask a doctor to prescribe Corning sunglasses with prescription lenses (find contact information in Appendix B). Corning lenses come in three shades of reddish amber. The lightest shade is best for most people, unless they are very light sensitive.

Corning lenses darken in sunlight. Lenses in the lightest shade stop about 50 percent of the light when worn indoors for contrast enhancement. When worn outdoors as sunglasses, they darken and stop 70 percent of the light, while still offering the contrast enhancement that helps so much. Many people complain that the medium and, especially, the darkest shades are too dark outdoors. Corning sunglasses cost about $300.

Ordinary sunglasses are available in an amber or yellow color. They can be found wherever sunglasses are sold. Avoid sunglasses in gray, smoke, or dark-green colors unless they are needed for extra light protection. These colors subdue color and contrast, thereby diminishing visual ability. The NOIR sunglasses mentioned in the preceding chapter are an amber color. A good choice for very light-sensitive persons are NOIR models 107 and 707; both are dark amber and provide contrast enhancement.

The manufacturer of NOIR sunglasses, Recreational Innovation (see Appendix B), also makes slightly tinted NOIR glasses for contrast enhancement indoors, in the same frame styles as listed in the preceding chapter. The difference is that these are for **indoor use only.** The model numbers are 711 and 111. The number 11 designates this lighter shade of amber. These are available with a prescription from New York Lighthouse for the Blind for about $13. Bossert Specialties sells them without a prescription for about $24.

The improvement in one's vision using contrast-enhancing lenses is often dramatic, especially when combined with other coping techniques. When used for reading, contrast enhancement adds the benefit of darkening the print on the page. Such an addition increases the improvement gained by using a magnifier. Contrast enhancement also helps one see television better. Video visual aids (see Chapter 22) do not photograph blue ink very well. Enhance the contrast by placing a sheet of amber or yellow cellophane or acetate over the print, and it will photograph as black.

There is a downside to wearing amber contrast-enhancing lenses: they alter perception of color. This is not a problem when amber lenses are used for driving. The red, amber, and green traffic signals are still easily identifiable. It's really an issue of aesthetics. Texas highways are bordered in spring by patches of wildflowers that are a joy to see. The red, yellow, and blue of these flowers could lighten anyone's day. Unfortunately, amber lenses convert Texas bluebonnets into "greenbonnets," indistinguishable from their green foliage. Red Indian paintbrushes are seen as off-white. Yellow flowers appear snow white. I miss seeing the wild explosion of color in the spring, but I still wear amber lenses. The added contrast improves my vision enough to make the sacrifice worthwhile.

CHAPTER 18

Talking Appliances and Large-Print Products

This book emphasizes vision rehabilitation, but there are times and situations when appliances that talk are beneficial. Examples of products available include talking calculators, watches, scales, blood-pressure monitors, and many more items. All of these products are also available with large-print displays. Bossert Specialties, LS&S, Maxi Aids, and Independent Living Aids all offer catalogs with large-print and talking products. The New York Lighthouse for the Blind has a catalog of nonoptical aids that are available without a prescription. See Appendix B for contact information.

There is a danger inherent in becoming dependent on talking appliances. An earlier chapter discussed the fact that we humans must **learn** how to see and that we can forget aspects of this skill, such as the ability to recognize printed words. When persons with visual impairment use equipment designed for the totally blind, they strengthen the tendency to forget what words look like. For this reason, use of talking products should be minimized, but occasional use shouldn't be a problem.

The public library has, or can borrow from other libraries, many books in large print for disabled readers. In addition, large-print books may be available without charge through the state library for the blind. Reader's Digest, Time magazine, and the New York Times Weekly are available in large print for a cost. Find contact information in Appendix B.

CHAPTER 19

Magnification: Make It Bigger

Disease	Usefulness (scale 1–10)	See note number
Cataracts	10	1
Diabetic retinopathy	10	1
Glaucoma	10	1
Macular degeneration	10	1
Retinitis pigmentosa	10	1

Scale

1 = Offers little if any help for someone with this disease.

4–5–6 = Moderately effective for someone with this disease.

10 = Very effective for someone with this disease.

(Other ratings can be gauged accordingly.)

Note

1. As long as a person has object vision, magnification is useful. If visual acuity drops to around 20/800 or less, optical magnification loses its effectiveness; but electronic magnifiers, like video visual aids, are still very effective. Persons with severe field loss may not profit from magnification.

Make It Bigger: A Basic Principle

The first coping technique I discussed was getting closer. Getting closer makes things look bigger through the principle of approach magnification. The limitations of approach magnification lie in the fact that the normal eye of an adult will not focus closer than four inches. People over age forty probably have accommodation problems (see Chapter 2), so their eyes may not focus closer than thirty-six inches.

To help the eye focus up close, the patient must use a lens, or magnifier. Bifocals are examples of magnifiers. Bifocals correct the inability to focus up close. They help the eyes to focus at sixteen inches. The magnifiers used by the visually impaired help the eye to focus at distances from less than one inch to about ten inches.

Almost all visually impaired persons try magnification at one time or another. This is logical. During the early stages of their disease, patients notice that they can read the newspaper headlines, but not the rest of the paper. Logically, if they could make all print the size of headlines, they could read the whole paper. Unfortunately, far too many patients find that magnifiers do not help. **If a magnifier does not work, one of four factors is involved:**

1. The patient is using his or her residual vision incorrectly. He or she is not using eccentric viewing or scanning.

2. He or she is using the magnifier incorrectly.

3. The magnifier is not strong enough.

4. The magnifier is possibly too strong, but this is rarely the case.

People buy magnifiers from office-supply stores or an optical company. They usually reject small magnifiers and choose a large one, because they think they will be able to see more at one time with it. **This is a mistake. Large magnifiers are weak.** By design, they have to be. A small magnifier may be weak, but a large one **must** be weak. Any magnifier four inches across will be no more than about +5 diopters (D.) or two-power (2X). A person with a visual acuity of 20/200 needs ten-power (10X). No wonder the large magnifier doesn't work!

Strong magnifiers are hard to find, but they are available up to +80 D. or 32X. A diopter (D.) is a unit of measurement of the refractive power of a lens. Two and a half diopters (D.) produce one-power (1X) of magnification. (If you are an eye-care professional and question this formula, please suspend judgment until you read the next chapter.)

How can someone with visual impairment find magnifiers strong enough for his or her needs? A low-vision specialist can supply them. Magnifiers appear in the recommended catalogs of visual aids, but proceed with caution. There are pitfalls in ordering one's own aids. Be sure to thoroughly understand the next two chapters before you do so.

CHAPTER 20

Low-Vision Aids and Their Use

The subject of low-vision aids is very broad; there is simply no way the topic can be covered completely. The best I can do is to introduce the subject. This chapter expands on the material in the preceding chapter, so the chart at the beginning of that chapter applies to this chapter too.

By definition, a low-vision aid is anything that helps a person with partial vision cope with his disability. This includes lane lines painted on highways, to mention only one example. Generally, however, the term "low-vision aid" refers to optical aids. Optical aids fall into two major categories. The more important category contains aids that help us to see up close (magnifiers); the other category contains aids that help us to see at a distance (telescopes).

Some telescopes and magnifiers are available to everyone through catalogs (nonprescription aids). Others are available only through an eye-care professional (prescription aids). Some low-vision specialists believe that all low-vision aids should be prescription aids. This is apparent in the policy of the New York Lighthouse for the Blind. They require a prescription for even a handheld magnifier. The general consensus does not support their policy, but I agree with them in principle, because of the frustrations low-vision patients often encounter when following the do-it-yourself method. It bears repeating: working with a good low-vision specialist is the surest way to discover the best solutions for one's particular problems and lifestyle. On the other hand, I believe that ordering one's own optical aids can be done successfully, if the reader exerts the effort to learn the basic facts presented in this book.

Low-Vision Optics

You should know a little about low-vision optics, even if you choose not to order aids for yourself. All persons with visual impairment need to understand certain terms.

Power and Diopters

The power of a lens is how much larger the lens makes an item appear. The symbol "X" here operates much like the multiplication sign. An 8X lens will make print one-eighth inch tall look as if it were one inch tall, or eight times larger.

The term "diopter" (D.) refers to the refractive power of a lens. It takes $+2\frac{1}{2}$ D. to produce a magnification power of 1X.

Eye-care professionals and manufacturers use a different formula. They say +4 D. = 1X. When a manufacturer says one of his magnifiers is 5X, he is saying it is +20 D. Four diopters times 5 equals +20 D. The problem with this formula is that it ignores approach magnification. A four-diopter lens focuses light ten inches behind the lens, and thus it does produce 1X. But when someone moves closer than ten inches, fewer diopters are required to make 1X, because approach magnification helps make things larger. In low-vision work, approach magnification is computed in the calculation, so that $+2\frac{1}{2}$ D. = 1X.

This formula is not much more accurate than the +4 D. formula. The closer one gets to the print, the fewer diopters he needs to produce 1X. At two to four inches, $2\frac{1}{2}$ D. may be about right to produce 1X. If one is working one-half inch from the print, two or even fewer diopters will produce 1X. The +4 D. formula is convenient for eye-care professionals. The $+2\frac{1}{2}$ D. formula is more accurate for low-vision applications, but it, too, is more convenient than accurate.

With this in mind, consider a +20 D. lens. The manufacturer calls it 5X, since he uses the +4 D. formula. When the $+2\frac{1}{2}$ D. formula is used, the result is 8X, a more accurate estimate of its power (+20 D. divided by $2\frac{1}{2} = 8X$).

Focal Length

Light passing through a positive (+) lens comes to a point of focus somewhere behind it. That distance is its focal length. By definition, a +1 D. lens focuses light at one meter. One meter equals about forty inches. The formula for determining the focal length of any lens is: forty divided by diopters equals focal length in inches. That is: 40/D. = inches. Therefore:

The focal length of a +10 D. lens = 40/10, or 4 inches.
The focal length of a +20 D. lens = 40/20, or 2 inches.
The focal length of a +40 D. lens = 40/40, or 1 inch.
The focal length of a +80 D. lens = 40/80, or $\frac{1}{2}$ inch.

Readers who understand the terms above will better understand the discussion of low-vision aids below.

Prescription Optical Aids

Prescription aids are available only through eye-care professionals. These are magnifiers or telescopes in spectacle form.

Magnifying Spectacles

There are two kinds of magnifying spectacles. The first type is a mass-produced pair of magnifying glasses in varying powers that a doctor can order from certain manufacturers. These will not contain the patient's prescription for nearsightedness, farsightedness, or astigmatism. The second type is a pair made to order for each patient, with his or her prescription ground in. The doctor begins with the patient's best prescription and then adds the amount of magnification needed to read a given size print.

There can be little argument that the latter is the superior aid. My experience indicates that doctors who dispense ready-made magnifying spectacles are less effective as low-vision specialists than those who do not. Ready-made glasses may be useful in training new patients or for temporary use until prescribed lenses are ready.

A typical person with macular degeneration might need glasses that are +20 D. This means the focal length of his lens will be two inches. The reading material must be held exactly two inches from the lens for it to be in sharp focus.

This introduces several concerns about using these glasses.

Using Magnifying Glasses

Since the focal length of magnifying glasses is so short (two inches in this example), the user cannot turn her head or eyes while reading. If the head is turned, the print will blur or disappear, because it is then farther than two inches from the lens. **Instead of turning the head or eyes to read, one must move the book.** Look straight ahead. Bring the book close until the print is in focus, then read along the line of print by moving the book to the left in front of the eye without moving the head or eye. Read one line, then track back to the left margin following the last line read. Drop down one line, then read the second line. This is the way to keep your place.

Patients can read with both eyes using spectacles in powers up to about +12 D. Spectacles stronger than this require using only one eye. When reading material must be held very close, both eyes cannot possibly see the same spot on the page.

When patients require more power than +12 D., doctors fit a magnifying lens for the better eye and block out the "off" eye. The best way to block out the off eye is to mount a lightweight lens that is heavily frosted. Some doctors use an occluder, an opaque plastic cover that clips over the lens of the off eye. These are a poor second choice.

Optometrists and some low-vision specialists are taught that glasses need to be balanced in weight. Some will fit patients with a clear +20 D. lens for the better eye and then use a frosted lens of equal power and weight for the off eye. They balance the glasses so they are weighted equally on both sides. This is totally unnecessary! It only adds weight to the glasses. For years I have worn +24 D. and +36 D. lenses for the left eye and a very lightweight frosted lens for the right eye with no balance problems of any kind.

Since the use of low-vision reading aids brings the patient very close to the material he is reading, using light correctly is critical. Review Chapter 16, "Light." It is crucial to hold the book so that light falls on it without shadows.

In 1986 I worked with a young man in Amarillo, Texas. He wore a baseball cap all the time. His magnifying glasses focused at two or three inches, so the bill of his cap got in the way. The bill held the reading material too far away from the glasses, and it also cast a dark shadow over the material. Finally, under protest, he took the cap off. This didn't help; his hair stuck out as far as the bill of his cap! This patient needed to modify his appearance to improve his visual ability. Other adjustments may also help. For example, I wear only clip-on ties and short-sleeved shirts. Regular ties that go around the neck and long sleeves both bind uncomfortably when I bend forward to use a magnifier.

Patients with blind spots anywhere in their central field of vision need to use eccentric viewing along with the magnifying glasses. Magnification makes the blind spot seem smaller, but it is still there. When a person with macular problems looks directly at a word through a magnifier, the blind spot will blot out a letter or two, or perhaps the whole word. To avoid this, fixate on the empty space between the line being read and the one above it. Do not fixate on the line of print you want to read.

Frames for Magnifying Glasses

The frames for magnifying lenses are very important. Apparently, many doctors, even some low-vision specialists, don't know this. The frames should be half-eye style. Some people call them "granny glasses" or "Ben Franklin" frames. Consider the situation. The lens prescribed for the better eye focuses at two inches. Anything not two inches from the lens cannot be seen. If full-size lenses are prescribed with the off eye frosted out, the glasses isolate the user from his surroundings.

The frames should allow the user to look over the lenses. This way, he stays in contact with his environment without having to remove the glasses to see something other than what he is reading. I have met people fitted with full-size magnifying lenses who, for this reason, rejected the glasses and refused to wear them.

Designs for Vision (see Appendix B) makes half-eye lenses up to +40 D. They make full-size lenses up to +80 D. Those who require the higher powers will have to be content with full-size lenses, but wherever possible, the half-eye frames should be used.

There are exceptions to this basic principle. The Volk Conoid lens made by Tech Optics is an exceptionally high-quality lens. (See Appendix B.) It is made of glass instead of plastic and is available in powers up to +100 D. It is available only in full-diameter lenses, not half-eye sizes. If a person has a choice of a Volk full-diameter lens or a half-eye style, after considering the issues involved, he may decide he prefers the full-diameter lens. This is fine, as long as he makes the choice after comparing the two lenses and understands the problem of isolation presented by the full-diameter lens. In this case, the user selects better image quality and accepts the limitations of the full-diameter lens.

There are two ways to make a magnifying lens. The first method is to include all the power in a single lens. The second method is to make two lenses and stack them together, creating a doublet. Up to about +18 D., single lenses are fine. Above +18 D., the doublet lens is a better choice. A +24 D. doublet is two +12 D. lenses stacked one on top of the other. The doublet lens will give a wider and deeper field of focus than a single lens of the same power.

Telescopic Glasses

Telescopic glasses are regular spectacles with a telescope glued to or through the regular lens. Figure 26.1, in Chapter 26, shows a typical pair. Telescopic glasses provide distance viewing, but supplemental lenses, called reading caps, are available to convert them for close viewing. Several manufacturers produce telescopic glasses. Keeler products are good; Walters are fine for classroom use; and there are others. These companies produce glasses according to doctors' specifications.

There are three basic configurations of telescopic glasses. The most common is the **spotting configuration** pictured in Figure 26.1. Here, the telescope is mounted in the upper segment of the carrier lens (that is, the lens containing, or carrying, the telescope), slanted up so that the chin must be lowered to see straight ahead through the scope. Most of the time the wearer looks through the carrier lens. The telescope is used briefly to spot distance objects. The spotting configuration is utilized in tasks like driving and reading blackboards in school. One telescope, instead of two, is the preferred format for these tasks.

The second is the **constant use configuration.** In this configuration, the telescope (or telescopes) is mounted in the very center of the carrier lens and points straight ahead. The eyes look through the scopes all the time. This configuration is used in tasks like watching TV, movies, and stage plays and in other tasks involving sitting and viewing distant objects. Using two telescopes in this configuration is more common.

The third type is called the **surgical configuration.** Surgeons with normal vision use these in performing delicate operations where magnification is needed. In this case, two scopes are mounted in the lower segment of the carrier lens, angled downward. Sometimes this configuration is useful for the visually impaired, for example, if the patient needs to see things below eye level. Some doctors fit the surgical configuration with close-up lenses for reading. While this gets the nose away from the book, patients pay a high price for the glasses in dollars and weight. The weight may be a greater deterrent than the dollars!

Two kinds of telescopic glasses are available. Full-diameter telescopes are almost as large as the carrier lens. The other type is smaller in diameter, such as those pictured in Figure 26.1. This chapter will be limited to discussing these smaller, more versatile telescopes, such as those made by Designs for Vision.

Mounting the smaller scope involves drilling a hole in the carrier lens. The telescope extends through the hole and is glued in place. This brings the scope very close to the eye and gives the widest field of view that the scope is capable of providing. Scopes glued to the outside of the carrier lens are farther from the eye and lose some of this important capability.

Besides variance in configuration, size, and power, there are two types of telescopes. A Galilean scope is a tube that contains at least two lenses spaced inside. Light travels straight through the tube. Prismatic or terrestrial telescopes are tubes also, but a prism inside bounces the light around before it comes out the other end.

Galilean scopes are less expensive and weigh less, but prismatic scopes provide a much wider field of view. The prismatic scopes focus from three feet to infinity. (Note: technically, twenty feet is infinity for the eye. This is why we use twenty feet in testing visual acuity. The shape of the lens inside the eye changes on targets out to twenty feet; after that there is no change in the shape of the lens, even on targets out millions of light years away, i.e., the stars. I use the term "infinity" here to mean "as far as the eye can see.")

Designs for Vision makes several Galilean scopes. Some are fixed-focus, while others are focusable. They offer the following powers of fixed-focus models: 1.7X, 2.2X, 2.2X wide-angle, 3.0X, 3.0X wide-angle, and 4.0X. Focusable models are available in 1.7X, 2.2X, 3.0X, and 4.0X. Both focusable and nonfocusable models are suitable for classroom use.

Designs for Vision provides the fixed-focus Galilean scopes with a focus +.12 D. short of infinity. This is ideal for classroom use, but Galilean scopes used for driving should be focused on infinity at the factory. The doctor must specify which is needed.

The 1.7X and 2.2X are the only two Galilean models I recommend for driving. All are suitable for classroom and other uses.

Most of the Galilean scopes are unsuitable for driving because of their very narrow field of view (recall that the field of view becomes narrower as the power goes up). Prismatic scopes in powers from 3X to 6X are better for driving. I drove with the 4X Galilean for nearly four years. I replaced it with the 6X prismatic that came out in 1976.

Prismatic scopes come in 2.5X, 3X, 4X, 5X, 6X, 7X, 8X, and 10X. These provide a wider field of view than the Galilean scopes of equal power. The 4X Galilean offers a $4\frac{1}{2}$-degree field, while the prismatic 4X offers a 9-degree field. All prismatic scopes are recommended for driving except the 7X, 8X, and 10X. The 6X currently produced provides a $6\frac{1}{2}$-degree field. My experience indicates that drivers need at least a 6-degree field.

All prismatic scopes are suitable for classroom use, but they are heavy; so a handheld monocular may prove more practical in some cases — and a lot cheaper as well.

Nonprescription Optical Aids

Many companies manufacture nonprescription optical aids. This is a multimillion-dollar business in the U.S. The visually impaired are willing to spend a lot of money to overcome vision loss.

Two kinds of nonprescription aids are available: aids for near viewing and aids for distant viewing.

Near or Reading Optical Aids

Reading aids come in many forms and powers. I have grouped them into basic types.

Head-Borne Magnifiers

Spectacles or glasses are head-borne, but the items labeled "head-borne magnifiers" in the nonprescription group do not include glasses.

Several types of head-borne magnifiers are available; most fall in the category of loupes. Jewelers use loupes to examine gemstones and watches. These usually attach to regular glasses and can be moved out of the way when not in use. The loupes normally used by the visually impaired come in powers from about +8 D. to +32 D.

Typically, loupes provide a very small field of view, even when compared to magnifying spectacles. Loupes work well and are inexpensive. Use loupes exactly like the magnifying spectacles discussed above.

Another head-borne magnifier is the Magnivisor (other brands have similar names; the word "visor" typically appears in the name). These are "hats" with a lens suspended in front of the eyes. Some of these have power ratings sufficient for low-vision use, but I don't recommend them. The lens is too far from the eye. Leave these to the normally sighted hobbyist who needs a little magnification.

Handheld Magnifiers

Handheld magnifiers are held in the hand above the material to be read. Most have handles. "Pocket" magnifiers have plastic or leather cases that serve as handles. Most are a single lens, but some are multiple lenses stacked together. Some include lights that are powered by batteries or can be plugged into a wall socket. Hundreds of models are available, in all shapes, sizes, and powers.

If a magnifier, lighted or not, is larger than two inches in diameter, it is probably unsuitable for persons with visual impairment.

Significant vision loss requires strong aids, and most such aids are smaller than two inches in diameter.

At a distance of sixteen inches, normal reading vision encompasses a circle only three-eighths inch in diameter. This sharp vision moves along the line, tracking the print. A person reading with a magnifier moves the magnifier instead of the eyes. When magnifiers are used correctly, the person probably sees more at one time through the magnifier than a person with normal vision sees with her own eyes. This fact is difficult for the partially sighted to accept, but it is true. Once the patient understands this principle and accepts it, she realizes she isn't as disabled as she thought.

Each magnifier has its own focal length, depending on its strength. A +20 D. magnifier, for example, focuses exactly two inches above the material being read. It cannot be held three inches above the text. It is in focus at two inches only. This requires a steady hand, and those who cannot hold it at a constant distance should consider "stand" magnifiers (see below).

The eye must also remain close to the magnifier. With a +20 D. lens, the eye should be about eight inches above the magnifier, or even closer. The stronger the magnifier, the closer the eye must be. I use a +53 D. magnifier for some things. This is so strong that my eye almost touches the lens. Remember that patients with low vision are combining the power of the lens with approach magnification. They need to get close, thereby maximizing approach magnification, even if the focal length of the lens does not require it.

Handheld magnifiers come in powers from +5 D. to +68 D. A clear-glass marble, incidentally, offers about +68 D. I know two people who are severely impaired who use clear glass marbles for magnifiers. One was studying to be a doctor! A marble produces distortion, so a commercially produced magnifier of the same power is preferable, but a lens will be about the same size. Bausch and Lomb makes a +68 D. magnifier that is about one-half inch in diameter. This provides a wider reading field than that seen by a person with normal vision. The difference is that a normally sighted person can view the material from a distance of sixteen inches, whereas a user who is visually impaired must be closer.

Persons with macular degeneration or with a disease that makes eccentric viewing profitable must use eccentric viewing with any magnifier. See Figure 20.1.

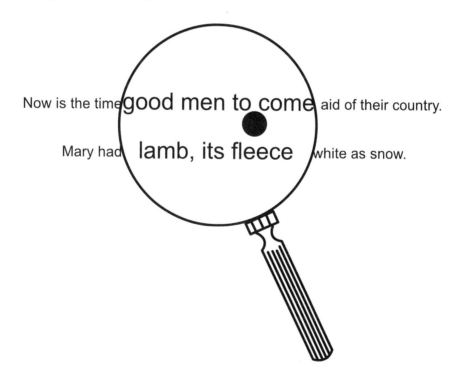

Now is the time good men to come aid of their country.

Mary had lamb, its fleece white as snow.

Figure 20.1: Using Eccentric Viewing with a Magnifier
Do not look directly at the word you want to read. Look above it or to the side of it. The black dot illustrates a typical point of fixation.

Stand Magnifiers

A stand magnifier is exactly what its name implies. It stands on the material to be read. Its base holds the lens at the proper focal length above the page.

This is the preferred magnifier for anyone whose hand is unsteady. Set the magnifier on the line to be read and slide it along the line of print. The stand holds the lens at the proper distance above the page, but the user must get his eye close enough to make it work correctly.

If the user is too far from the lens, he sees only a small field under the magnifier. For example, he might see only one letter at a time. With the eye close, he can see everything inside the circle of the magnifier's stand. With a +20 D. lens, move to within eight inches of the lens. If the lens is stronger, get even closer.

People often have problems reading a thermostat using a stand magnifier the conventional way. This happens because the indicator one needs to see in a thermostat is under a piece of glass below the focal point of the lens. To read a thermostat, turn the stand magnifier upside down. Put the base against the eye, and then lean close to the thermostat until the needle comes into focus.

Lighted Stand Magnifiers

Lighted stand magnifiers are stand magnifiers that include a light source. Some are battery-operated, while others plug into a wall outlet. This is generally the preferred magnifier for persons with macular problems. They need light and often need a way to hold the magnifier steady.

People who are photophobic can wear their sunglasses while reading with a lighted magnifier. The NOIR 01 amber color is excellent for this use. The amber lenses increase contrast, making the print darker on the page while protecting eyes from the glare.

Desk-Mounted Lighted Magnifiers

Because of their relatively large size, devices of this type can provide only low-power magnification. Do not buy one unless your disease has stabilized and will not get worse. I advised my mother not to buy one, but she did anyway, and now it sits in a closet, unused. Typically, these contain +5 D. lenses four inches or more across. Most have a built-in circular light. They sit on the floor or desk, or clamp to its edge. Some have a smaller, more powerful lens ground into the larger, weaker lens.

If one's visual acuity is 20/60 or better, these may be of use. But patients with a progressive disease will find that they become useless in a short time. I have seen hundreds of them sitting unused because they are not strong enough. My mother, who had AMD, used hers only a month.

Telescopic Aids

Telescopic aids are for viewing things at a distance. This group includes binoculars, monoculars (for one eye), and sport glasses. I know a man who attended college wearing his father's large navy binoculars around his neck. They enabled him to read the blackboard. (He also invented the first video visual aid.) Binoculars are fine, but monoculars are smaller, lighter, and far more portable. Most of the miniature monoculars are only three to four inches long.

While the consumer cannot trust the power rating on magnifiers (see Chapter 21, "How Much Magnification?" for a brief discussion of this issue), he can generally trust the rating on telescopic aids. It is helpful to know how these devices are rated. Their ratings have two numbers, for example, 7X35, 8X50, or 10X30.

The first number indicates **power.** Things seen through this device will appear larger (or closer) by a factor of seven times, or eight times, or ten times, to use the preceding examples. Stated another way, objects seen through this device will be enlarged by a factor equal to this number.

The power of a scope determines how well a person sees through it. If a user with a visual acuity of 20/120 looks through a 4X scope, she will see things with a visual acuity of 20/30 (120 divided by 4 equals 30). (The power of a magnifier — when computed with the 2 1/2 D. rule — affects vision the same way. A 10X, or +25D., lens permits a person with a visual acuity of 20/200 to read 20/20 size print: 200 divided by 10 equals 20.)

The second number in the rating refers to the size in millimeters of the larger front lens on the scope. Thirty-five means that the scope's front lens is thirty-five millimeters in diameter. The diameter of the lens relates to the light-gathering ability of that scope. A 7X20 scope would provide seven power, but it would not be as bright as a 7X35 scope.

Do not confuse the size of the lens as having any relationship to the scope's field of view. Recall that field of view is a function of the lens's power, as stated in the first number of the scope's rating. The more powerful the scope, the narrower the area seen at any given distance. Sometimes field of view is more important than the ability to see detail. In that case, select less power to have a larger field. If seeing detail is more important than field of view, select the stronger aid.

On all telescopic devices, there is a point inside which the scope will not focus. An 8X scope, for example, might not focus inside sixteen feet. The stronger the telescope, the farther away this point will be.

Many telescopic devices are available with supplemental lenses that bring their focal distance closer. Any scope is convertible to "near use" by adding a positive lens to the end of the scope. For example, with my driving telescopic glasses, I use a +2.75 D. lens to read the speedometer. The power of the reading cap controls the new focal length of the scope.

Some telescopic devices come in "near focus" models. The 8X20 Selsi, model 164, is a good example. It focuses on objects from eleven inches to infinity with no supplemental lens required. This is a highly versatile aid. I use one for reading the descriptive material next to artifacts inside museum exhibit cases. It is equally useful for viewing more distant objects. Walters makes an 8X20 model almost identical to the Selsi 164.

Sport glasses are binoculars mounted in spectacle frames. Persons with normal vision use them at football games and other sporting events. They come in powers from 2.5X to 10X. Opera glasses, by comparison, are usually 3X. Opera glasses are handheld, but they will also work well.

Sport glasses are very useful for persons with low vision. Typical uses for them are watching movies, TV, and stage plays, and viewing scenery while **riding** in a car. **Never use sport glasses for driving.** Sport glasses obscure one's peripheral vision, so driving with them would be like driving with tunnel vision. (Later in the book I discuss the fact that some visually impaired persons can drive with telescopic glasses. These telescopic glasses, specifically built for this purpose, do not obscure peripheral vision.) All of these viewing tasks — such as watching movies, TV, and stage plays, and viewing scenery — can be enjoyed with less than 20/20 vision. A patient with 20/200 vision wearing 4X sport glasses will have a visual acuity through the scopes of 20/50. This improvement in visual acuity is enough to enjoy these activities. While sport glasses of any power are helpful to persons with normal vision at sports events, those with a power of 4X or less are not effective for the visually impaired. At a football game, for example, the user is too far from the action for them to be of much help. Beecher brand scopes (listed in Appendix B) offer sufficient power to be helpful, but in the higher powers, the field of view is so small they lose much of their effectiveness.

All telescopic devices provide a given field of view that is far smaller than the human eye's. If someone goes to a movie with sport glasses and sits close to the screen, he sees so little of the screen that he misses much of the action. If he sits in the back, he sees more of the screen at one time, but he may not see it very well. One must compromise clarity and field width. Experience will soon indicate what works best for each individual. When sitting in the front, back, or middle, one must move the head to follow the action on the screen. When watching television with sport glasses, one must sit close enough so that the screen completely fills the view through the scopes. See Chapter 27, on watching TV, for more information about sport glasses.

Persons with macular degeneration, and others who profit by using eccentric viewing, should use the following technique when using telescopic devices. Aim the scope at what you wish to see, then look through the scope, pointing your eyes to the side of the target. See Figure 20.2.

Nonoptical Aids

The list of nonoptical aids is almost endless. This discussion touches on only a few of them.

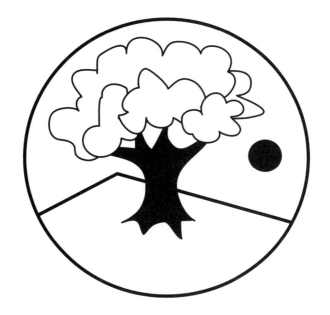

Figure 20.2: Using Eccentric Viewing with a Telescope
The black dot is a typical point of fixation.

Examples of nonoptical aids include felt-tip pens that make a broad, bold line more easily seen by the visually impaired than the line produced by standard pens. There are bookstands that hold the book at eye level, allowing one to get close without bending down. Big-button telephones, large-number cooking timers, needle threaders, and countless other household items exist that make life easier for the visually impaired. Browse through the catalogs recommended in Appendix B.

Wide-line paper — with lines spaced much further apart than normal — makes writing easier. You can order wide-line paper from the American Printing House for the Blind (see Appendix B). For years, I've used wide-line paper that I designed myself and have printed by a local printer. See an example in Figure 20.3. The

Figure 20.3: Wide-Line Paper
Designed for use with a video visual aid. The wide right margin warns the user he is about to run off the page.

first time I did this, I used a typewriter to prepare the original, but a computer will work just as well. Set the machine on double space, or triple space if preferred. Use the underline key to make lines on the page.

Take the original to a print shop or to a photocopy retailer such as Kinko's to have multiple copies made. The print quality will be higher if you use a print shop, but photocopying will probably be cheaper. The print shop or the photocopy shop can put the paper into tablet form at little additional cost. Students might wish to order copies with holes punched for loose-leaf notebooks. For my purposes, the wide-line paper I've developed is better than what is available through the American Printing House.

If you write with a video visual aid, consider having paper printed that has a wider margin on the right than on the left. When writing with a video visual aid, it is easy to lose track of where one is on the page. The wide right margin warns the user he is about to run off the page. Again, see Figure 20.3.

CHAPTER 21

How Much Magnification?

This chapter tells you how to compute the amount of magnification you need when purchasing magnification devices. Many readers will simply want to skip ahead to the next chapter.

I hesitated including this information because it gives people the ability to order their own magnifiers. The danger in ordering your own magnifiers lies in the fact that manufacturers do not always label their magnifiers accurately. Why this is the case is a hard question to answer. I've heard a theory that one manufacturer of magnifiers apparently assumes the user will read with the magnifier while wearing bifocals, and therefore the company labels the magnification of its products accordingly. I've heard that another company apparently assumes the eye has the ability to produce one power of magnification. Both or neither of these may be true, and there may be other explanations. Whatever the explanation, one reputable manufacturer labels a stand magnifier +28 D. when it is only +17.6 D. Another is labeled +20 D. when it is only +9 D. Another, made by the same company, is labeled +20 D., and it is indeed +20 D. The inconsistency in labeling aids creates problems for those who do not know the actual power of aids they buy. I repeat: the visually impaired need the help of a low-vision specialist. Only rarely should patients order their own aids.

On the other hand, understanding how to compute magnification is good knowledge to possess — if used responsibly.

STEP ONE: Refer to the section in Chapter 1 titled "Testing Your Visual Acuity." Obtain the most accurate reading possible, in feet, of how far you are from the chart when all three numbers are readable. Those with macular problems must use eccentric viewing while reading the numbers. If you will be wearing glasses while using a magnifier, use the glasses when taking this test. Patients who have given up their glasses because they don't help much, and who will not be using them while working with a magnifier, should leave them off during this test.

STEP TWO: Determine your visual acuity. The letters on the chart are the 100-foot size, so the denominator — or second number — of your visual acuity is 100. The numerator — or first number — is the distance in feet you were standing from the chart when all three numbers were readable. Consider the following simple example: if all three numbers on the chart were readable at 10 feet, and the letter size is 100, then the visual acuity is 10/100.

STEP THREE: Solve the following simple math problem. The formula to compute how much magnification you need is as follows: The reciprocal — or inverse — of one's visual acuity equals the diopters needed to read textbook-size print.

Therefore, the reciprocal of visual acuity 10/100 is 100/10, which equals +10 D.

STEP FOUR: If you are over forty or have ever worn bifocals, add five more diopters.

+10 D. plus +5 D. = +15 D.

If this hypothetical person uses a +15 D. lens, he should be able to read Jaeger 5 print (textbook-size print).

To read small print, like Jaeger 2 (the ability to read Jaeger 2 at 16 inches indicates 20/20 vision), another step is involved. Start with the number of diopters obtained from Step Three above. In the example above, this was +10 D. Multiply this by $2\frac{1}{2}$:

+10 D. x $2\frac{1}{2}$ = +25 D.

Now add the +5 D. for being over age forty or having worn bifocals, and get +30 D.

A +30 D. lens should give the person in this example the ability to read Jaeger 2, which is the equivalent of the small print readable by persons with normal vision from a distance of sixteen inches.

The formulas stipulate that the reciprocal of one's visual acuity **in diopters** provides the ability to read Jaeger 5, or 50-size print. The reciprocal of visual acuity **in power** (that is, multiplied by $2\frac{1}{2}$) gives the diopters needed to read Jaeger 2, or small print. In each case, when there are accommodation problems, as indicated by the need for bifocals or being over age forty, add +5 D. more.

The purpose of this exercise is to determine where to begin **reality testing.** The formula works well, although it works better when one's near visual acuity is used rather than one's distance acuity. In either case, sometimes it proves wrong. The final proof is in reality testing. In other words, try the lens indicated to determine whether it permits you to read a given size print. You may find that the computations have resulted in your selecting an aid that is not strong enough or even one that is too strong. This is why it is essential to order aids only from companies that allow customers to return unwanted merchandise.

CHAPTER 22

Video Visual Aids

Disease	Usefulness (scale 1–10)	See note number
Cataracts	10	1
Diabetic retinopathy	10	1
Glaucoma	7–8–9	1
Macular degeneration	10	1
Retinitis pigmentosa	7–8–9	1

Scale

1 = Offers little if any help for someone with this disease.

4–5–6 = Moderately effective for someone with this disease.

10 = Very effective for someone with this disease.

(Other ratings can be gauged accordingly.)

Note

1. Even after object and travel vision are gone, a "patch" of retinal tissue may function well enough to use video visual aids.

What Is a Video Visual Aid?

Doctors often do not show video visual aids to patients during the first few appointments. There is a good reason for this. They want patients to develop other skills first. Video visual aids are too easy.

They provide instant vision rehabilitation. If this is a person's only aid, it handicaps him or her. He or she may not expend the effort to learn to use other aids.

The visually impaired face a fundamental problem. They can't read. Reading is the basic survival skill in Western society. A video visual aid provides reading ability while one is sitting in front of it, but as soon as she walks away, she is blind again. To survive and compete in society, the visually impaired must be able to read no matter where they are. This means they must always carry an aid in their pocket or purse, and video visual aids will not fit in a pocket or purse. These machines are a convenience to those who can afford them, but they must be only one among many aids.

The video visual aid is the reading aid of choice for people with visual acuities around 20/800 or worse. All patients with macular degeneration can use them for the rest of their lives, even if they live to be 150. Persons with diabetic retinopathy and retinitis pigmentosa can use them long after they have lost all travel vision and most object vision. Even in such severe cases of vision loss, there usually remains a patch of retinal tissue that allows the person to use eccentric viewing and thus read with these machines.

Around 1968, an engineer named Dr. Sam Genensky (who is legally blind) experimented with closed-circuit television (CCTV) as a reading aid for the partially sighted. He found it exceptionally helpful. From this beginning emerged a new commercial product made by various manufacturers. Telesensory, Seeing Technology, Humanware, and Optelec are the leading manufacturers today. Contact any of them for a free, no obligation demonstration in your home or office. (Find contact information in Appendix B.) Distributors who refuse to come to the home of a prospective customer are not likely to serve the customer's needs after the sale.

These reading machines comprise a small TV camera connected to a TV monitor (basically, a TV set), with a moving table under the camera. Reading material is placed on this platform, which is moved back and forth under the camera. The camera photographs the material, enlarges it up to sixty times the original size, and displays the enlarged print on the TV screen. With these machines, many people with a true visual acuity of 20/6000 — or even worse — can still read.

A twelve-inch-screen model is large enough for most purposes. Larger screens offer little additional benefit, except in installations where two cameras are used. One camera displays the platen of a typewriter, while the other photographs the draft copy. The screen is split so that both images appear on the same screen.

Prices for video visual aids run from $1,800 to $3,500. Some states do not charge sales tax on these machines if the patient has a prescription from a doctor for a video visual aid. In addition, the cost of the machines is deductible from federal income tax as a medical expense or as a business machine, if that can be justified. Medicare and some insurance companies have been known to pay for them, but only after long legal hassles.

Video visual aids have changed greatly in recent years. In 1990 almost all were black-and-white models. Today, all companies make them in color. The color models always include a black-and-white capability. Color offers no advantage over the black-and-white models, and most people will see the black and white better because of greater contrast. For these reasons, color machines are recommended only for persons with jobs that require color discrimination. Obviously, the salesman would prefer to sell you the higher-priced color machine.

All video visual aids provide writing capability, and some feature typing accessories for use on typewriters that have a moving platen. The camera sees only a small part of the platen, so moving-ball typewriters will not work. The typewriter sits under the camera, and the user sees what he is typing on the screen. The user does not see the keyboard, so touch-typing is required. When used for writing, the hand and tablet go under the camera. The user looks at the screen instead of at his hand. At first this feels awkward, but most people quickly learn that seeing one's hand on the screen is the same as seeing it on the desk. Both the hand and the tip of the pen are visible on the screen, permitting the user to see how to shape the letters. Figure 22.1 shows a video visual aid in use.

Figure 22.1: A Video Visual Aid, or Closed-Circuit Television Reading Machine

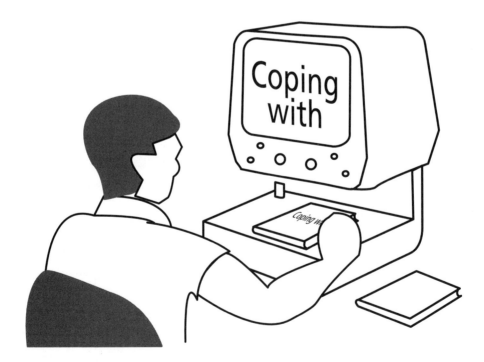

Proper Use of Video Visual Aids

Video visual aids provide instant vision rehabilitation, but proper use enhances their effectiveness.

The machines have a positive and a negative mode. The positive image presents black letters on a white background. The negative image presents white letters on a black background. The negative image makes reading easier. At first it will seem strange, but the eye sees white letters on a black background better than it sees black letters on a white background.

Make the print on the screen larger than necessary. Don't struggle with print that is too small or hard to read. As magnification increases, less material shows on the screen. This doesn't matter. Do not place print on the screen and then read across it. Instead, fixate on one spot on the screen and let the print pass by that spot. Do not move your head or eyes. Move only your hands.

Chapter 4 discussed how concentration can short-circuit the blinking reflex, causing the eyes to dry out and hurt. **You can solve this problem.** Blink after reading the first line of print and continue to blink deliberately to lubricate the eyeballs and keep them moist.

After reading the first line, push the moving table to the right, tracking the line of print last read. This prevents losing one's place. As you do this, blink again. Then push the moving table forward. This moves the next line of print to the middle of the screen. Do this with each line. Do not read a whole screen full of material before moving the table up. Read only the line of print in the center of the screen. Ignore other print that also may appear on the screen.

Those who need eccentric viewing to see best must use it here. Look above or to the side of words, but don't look very far off to the side. At this reading distance, the blind spot for those with macular problems is very small. Normally the point of fixation will be a spot between the line being read and the one above it. Persons with diabetic retinopathy and retinitis pigmentosa may need to fixate farther from the word they want to see.

Remember, keep your head and eyes still. Look at one spot on the screen.

CHAPTER 23

Elvis and Jordy

The LVES system (pronounced Elvis) and Jordy glasses provide electronic approaches to solving vision problems. LVES stands for Low Vision Enhancement System. Jordy glasses take their name from the character in "Star Trek: The Next Generation" who wears funny-looking glasses.

These systems are not for everyone, and they are relatively expensive. In April 2000, Jordy glasses cost $2,795 **wholesale** plus up to $250 more for optional equipment. Retail distributors typically increase the price and may charge additional fees for training.

The LVES system is in transition. The first firm that manufactured it has dropped the product. Another manufacturer (Beta-Com, a Canadian company) plans to begin production of the second-generation model during 2001, with a projected wholesale cost of $2,500. In the past, the LVES system was fitted only at certain locations; a three-day training session cost over $1,000. How the new policy will work has yet to be determined. At this writing, first-generation LVES systems are still available at greatly reduced prices.

The LVES system and Jordy glasses operate on the same principle. One or more subminiature TV cameras, built into the glasses or headset, photograph near or distant objects and display the magnified image on a small TV screen, also built into the glasses or headset. Theoretically, a person with a visual acuity of 20/480 should be able to read a newspaper with either product. The new

LVES model will be in color, will weigh less, and will cost less —
three features the first-generation LVES lacks. Jordy is also in color.

Neither system is, or even looks, like conventional glasses. The
only similarity is that they fit on one's head. There are no lenses to
look through. You are actually looking into an opaque box, seeing
only what is displayed on the small screens in front of your eyes.
Both systems are useful only for sitting tasks. They are not worn for
driving or for walking around.

The systems are powered by a battery pack worn on the waist.
The battery must be recharged every two to three hours. This is
one of the shortcomings, but more than one battery pack can be
carried to keep the system operational. Both systems will work at
home from an AC adapter. At extra cost, Jordy is available with a
battery allowing four hours of use. The new LVES will surely offer
the same feature.

I know only one person who has purchased one of these
systems. He is displeased with it on two counts. He cannot read his
computer screen with it because the image appears too blurred,
and the battery never lasts more than thirty minutes. (I suspect
that his particular unit may not be working properly.)

These systems can be described as viewing a sixty-inch television set from about six feet away. In other words, one's field of
vision is restricted. Normal vision provides fields of about 120
degrees vertically and 180 degrees horizontally. These products
provide about 50 degrees vertically and 40 degrees horizontally.
The restricted field makes the system unsuitable for driving or
walking. Some readers might wonder why, as patients drive with
telescopic glasses that provide only a 6- to 13-degree field. The
difference is that with the LVES and Jordy systems, the user sees
only the 50- by 40-degree field. All peripheral vision is gone.
Whereas, when using the telescope for driving, the patient drives

most of the time using his full field of vision. The telescope is used only occasionally, not all the time, and even when it is used, one's peripheral vision is still functional.

The LVES and Jordy systems are designed to improve visual acuity. They may be inappropriate for persons who have lost field vision, but I cannot make that determination. Interested persons should discuss their vision problems with the suppliers to determine applicability.

The LVES system was developed by Johns Hopkins University, NASA, and the Veterans Administration. For more information and fitting locations, contact the Wilmer Low Vision Clinic. For information about Jordy glasses, contact the manufacturer, Enhanced Vision Systems. Contact information for both organizations is given in Appendix B.

CHAPTER 24

Aids for the Computer User

Disease	Usefulness (scale 1–10)	See note number
Cataracts	10	1
Diabetic retinopathy	10	1
Glaucoma	7–8–9	1
Macular degeneration	10	1
Retinitis pigmentosa	7–8–9	1

Scale

1 = Offers little if any help for someone with this disease.

4–5–6 = Moderately effective for someone with this disease.

10 = Very effective for someone with this disease.

(Other ratings can be gauged accordingly.)

Note

1. Video visual aids were once used to photograph computer screens. These products have been replaced by newer technology. The picture quality is better than video, and any person who can use a video visual aid can also use the products discussed in this chapter.

Reading Aids and Voice Aids

Special software is available to enlarge print and graphics on computer screens. Sometimes this software creates problems for computers in a network; there should be no problem with stand-alone computers. The following products enable the visually impaired to read a computer screen. These products enlarge print on the screen up to two or three inches tall. Print size is adjustable. People with a visual acuity as low as 20/6000 or worse can usually use them. Test a product before buying it, or make sure you have return privileges if it is ordered from a catalog.

Telesensory's Vista is a good product, and it ought to be, with a price tag of $2,495! (Find Telesensory in Appendix B.) Many other brands are available, and all are less expensive than Vista. Similar products appear in the catalogs this book recommends. Carefully study the description of each product for needed features and hardware requirements.

In my opinion, one of the best bargains is an enlarging program called Magic (which stands for MAGnification In Color). Contact Bossert Specialties for more information (see Appendix B). The price is about $350, subject to change, of course. I add a special cautionary note about Magic. I bought and use Version 2.0. It works fine. Since that purchase, the company has sent me versions 6.0 and 6.1. I tried and rejected 6.0 and 6.1 because they repeatedly locked up my computer. I dumped them and reinstalled my old version 2.0. I have also heard good reports on a product called Zoomtext.

Large-print stick-on labels affixed to the keys of the keyboard help the partially sighted computer user. These come in both black letters on a white background and white letters on a black background. The latter works best for most users. The letters and numbers are large and bold, and there are labels for special keys. The labels are plastic and quite durable. A set is available from LS&S Group for about $25. The New York Lighthouse Consumer Catalog offers a set for $10 that is basically the same product as the one sold by LS&S.

Some computer users might consider painting special keys on the keyboard with a bright color to make them stand out. Airplane-model dope (paint) works well, but first clean the keys with a cloth moistened with alcohol.

Today, voice synthesizers can be added to a computer's software package to make a computer talk. Voice-recognition software is also available that allows the user to give the computer voice commands and to dictate text. Voice-recognition software that will also speak the text that is on the screen costs about $500. Inquire about Microsoft's Speech, Dictation, and Voice software. MS Voice allows the user to give voice commands, such as "Start Microsoft Word," to the computer. MS Dictation allows the user to dictate letters or other text into the computer. Despite decades of research in this field, the accuracy rate for transcribing voice into text on the screen remains at 90 to 95 percent. The software has provisions for correcting these mistakes.

When my vision was 20/120, I used a computer successfully with a special work-area modification. A platform was built to hold the monitor at eye level and bring it closer to my face. A small fluorescent-light fixture was mounted under this shelf to illuminate the keyboard. I used glasses with +18 D. lenses to read the screen. Since the screen was at eye level and near my eyes, I could see it without bending severely, despite the two-inch focal length of the glasses.

The spectacles worked well, but later they were improved. Originally, to look down to find a specific key, I had to remove the glasses. I had another pair made, containing an +18 D. lens for the left eye that looked straight ahead. The right lens was frosted out. In the lower half of the frames, lenses like bifocals were mounted that focused on the keyboard.

Help for the Moderately Impaired

Several other possibilities exist for those with only modest visual impairment. None of the following methods will help patients with significant loss.

The standard screen used with computers measures about fifteen inches. Substituting a nineteen-inch screen makes the print on the screen two times larger. Monitors are available with screens even larger than nineteen inches. The larger the screen, the larger the print.

The Macintosh computer includes a feature to enlarge the print. Let a dealer demonstrate it for you. Microsoft Windows also includes a feature to enlarge print on the screen. Some, but not all, features in Windows allow you to select the size font you wish to use.

Those using DOS-based software might try using the DOS MODE command to change from an eighty-column display to forty. To do this, type in MODE 40 from a C:\ prompt. This command can also be placed in your autoexec.bat file so that it is executed each time you turn on the computer. This will increase print size on the screen.

A good resource for people who want to further explore the options available to them is <u>Computer and Web Resources for People with Disabilities, Third Edition</u> by the Alliance for Technology Access (Alameda, CA: Hunter House, 2000).

I have recommended using a combination of aids or coping techniques. Try one of these techniques in combination with a larger monitor.

CHAPTER 25

Special Aids for Field Loss

Disease	Usefulness (scale 1–10)	See note number
Cataracts	1	1
Diabetic retinopathy	1	1
Glaucoma	8–9–10	1
Macular degeneration	1	1
Retinitis pigmentosa	8–9–10	1

Scale

1 = Offers little if any help for someone with this disease.

4–5–6 = Moderately effective for someone with this disease.

10 = Very effective for someone with this disease.

(Other ratings can be gauged accordingly.)

Note

1. The effectiveness of aids discussed in this chapter depends on visual acuity and how much field vision remains. See the text for more details.

Vision Expanders

When a person looks through a pair of binoculars, the scope brings objects closer, but he sees only a narrow field. Looking through a scope backward produces the opposite effect. He sees a much wider field, but items will appear smaller by a factor equal to the power of the scope. For example, a 4X scope when used backward will reduce items seen by a factor of four, but it produces a much wider field of view.

Doctors use this principle to give patients with retinitis pigmentosa and glaucoma who have developed tunnel vision a wider field of view. If a patient's problem is mostly field loss and not visual acuity, this approach can prove helpful. Low-vision specialists often use the criterion that the patient needs a visual acuity of at least 20/40 before they prescribe these aids. I disagree with this rule. It is the patient's right to try any aid and decide for himself or herself whether it is appropriate and worth the cost.

The Designs for Vision 2.2X Galilean scope is a good vision expander when mounted in glasses **backward**. The scope reduces the size of objects seen through it by a factor of 2.2, so one's visual acuity drops accordingly. If a patient's visual acuity is 20/20, the scope will reduce it to 20/44.

20/30 will become 20/66
20/40 will become 20/88
20/50 will become 20/110
20/60 will become 20/132
20/80 will become 20/176
20/100 will become 20/220

Even in this last example, a visual acuity of 20/220 is better than mine, and better than that needed for independent mobility.

If one's visual acuity is in this range, and the field vision is less than 10 degrees, this scope would provide better mobility vision. Reduced visual acuity is preferable to severe field loss. Glasses like this do not permit reading, but for mobility, the field of view through the 2.2X scope mounted backward is about 20 degrees.

A patient can easily determine if this aid might help. Most

good low-vision specialists have this scope. Ask to try it. It doesn't need to be mounted in glasses. Simply hold the scope to the eye backward and observe the results. I am not suggesting that the low-vision specialist and his or her expertise be ignored. This test should provide enough data to help you decide whether you want to invest in further testing and fitting by specialists.

Other aids for field expansion are the Ocutech Image Minifier and the Ocutech Field Viewer. Both use the same principle as the 2.2X Galilean scope. The first, mounted in spectacles, makes either a monocular or binocular system. The second is a handheld aid. A low-vision specialist can obtain either from the Optical Aids Division of the New York Lighthouse.

Night Scopes

Night scopes, which help a person to see in the dark, are prescription aids sold only by certain eye-care professionals. For those afflicted with night blindness, such as persons with retinitis pigmentosa, these aids are sometimes useful for independent travel at night. Most are handheld; looking through them, everything appears in green light. They usually cost $2,000 or more; occasionally one can be found for around $400.

Boat owners sometimes use night scopes to dock their boats at night. Inquiries at a marina might locate one to try. Again, I don't mean you should bypass the expertise of the low-vision specialist. Trying a night scope is simply a way to collect data to make a decision whether to spend money for professional help in prescribing the aid. Contact Bossert Specialties for more information, prices, and a source of supply. The RP Foundation can also provide sources. See Appendix B.

CHAPTER 26

Aids for Driving

Disease	Usefulness (scale 1–10)	See note number
Cataracts	4–5–6	1
Diabetic retinopathy	4–5–6	1
Glaucoma	1–2–3	1
Macular degeneration	4–5–6	2
Retinitis pigmentosa	1–2–3	1

Scale

1 =   Offer little if any help for someone with this disease.

4–5–6 = Moderately effective for someone with this disease.

10 =   Very effective for someone with this disease.

(Other ratings can be gauged accordingly.)

Notes

1. Driving requires field vision more than visual acuity. This restricts persons with RP and glaucoma from using telescopic aids to drive. New York state, for example, requires a 140-degree field of vision.

2. Most persons with macular degeneration could drive with telescopic glasses if vision were the only variable in driving. Poor coordination and reflexes, impaired mobility, and rigidity often prevent people over sixty-five from driving, even when telescopic glasses improve their vision.

A Raging Controversy

This chapter is an introduction to the subject of driving with telescopic glasses (sometimes called bioptic glasses). Part V of this book contains more information for those who desire to pursue this subject in more depth.

I have already stated that I drive with telescopic glasses. Thousands of people do. Some doctors have opposed their use for driving. A battle royal is being waged out there between the pros and the cons on this subject.

Because of this dispute, some states have made the glasses illegal for driving. Other states license people with them. Still other states have no law either for or against their use, but by policy do or do not license people with them. It is primarily ophthalmologists who oppose telescopic glasses for driving, and their opposition clearly accents their poor understanding of subnormal vision.

To Try or Not to Try

Should you try to obtain a driver's license? This is a tough question, and it takes real soul-searching to do the right thing. Driving is something most persons with visual impairment want to do.

Low-vision specialists who prescribe telescopic glasses for driving generally estimate that only 6 to 10 percent of persons with visual impairment are candidates for driving. I agree with these figures, if the total population of the visually impaired is considered. If only those under age fifty are considered, the percentage is much higher.

Vision is not the only factor to consider in driving safely. Other limiting factors are coordination, reflexes, and mobility. I once told a ninety-two-year-old man he shouldn't try for a license. "Well, why not?" he snarled. "You do it, so why can't I?"

I responded, "Sir, when you can go out there in the front yard and turn a handspring, I'll work with you and try to get you licensed." So help me, this elderly man who was severely crippled with arthritis struggled to his feet and headed for the front door. He was going out there to prove he could turn a handspring! I knew exactly how he felt and sympathized with him, but I felt grateful when his wife interceded and helped me get him back on the sofa.

If one's agility and reflexes are good, if there are no crippling conditions present, and if money one can risk losing is available, the patient might try for a license using telescopic glasses.

First, learn whether your state licenses people with telescopic glasses. Most low-vision specialists prescribe them. Most of these doctors are highly ethical; if they feel it is unwise to fit a person with them, they will refuse to do so.

Telescopic glasses cost $500 to $2,500. The cost depends on the doctor's fee structure, the type and power of the scope used, and whether the doctor prescribes one or two scopes. The patient wishing to try for a license must have money that he or she can risk losing. The doctor cannot guarantee that the state medical-advisory board will issue a license, so the patient might purchase this expensive product only to be denied the license. All the doctor can do is ensure that one's visual acuity through the scope meets state requirements. When the state receives this and other data, officials decide on the individual case. They either issue a license or deny the application.

As a rule, it is a waste of time to ask officials if they will license a person before buying the glasses. In most states, the patient must risk buying the glasses, and then apply for the license. Note, however, that a low-vision specialist can determine whether or not your visual acuity through the scope is sufficient to meet state requirements before you buy the glasses.

Using Telescopic Glasses: Some Basics

Learning to use telescopic glasses properly is essential, but doing so is difficult for some people. Part V of this book contains more of the information one needs to know. Additionally, a self-directed training program is included for learning to use the glasses correctly.

When driving with telescopic glasses, the user does not look through the telescope all the time. Ninety percent of the time, the user drives without the scope. A bioptic user must trust his diminished vision and learn to use it correctly.

Notice in Figure 26.1 how the scope is tilted upward. The user lowers the chin to level the scope momentarily to see straight ahead. The user then raises the chin, lifting the scope out of the way. Moderately good reflexes and coordination are required to switch back and forth quickly from use of the eyes alone to use of the scope.

The scope is used to read signs, see traffic lights, and see farther down the street than a visually impaired person can see with his or her own eyes. When the driver isn't looking through the telescopic lens, he or she is looking through the carrier lens that holds the scope. The driver will see things down the road he cannot identify using his own eyes. He then uses the scope to spot and identify these "unknowns." **Those with macular problems must also use eccentric viewing to get their blind spot above the road.**

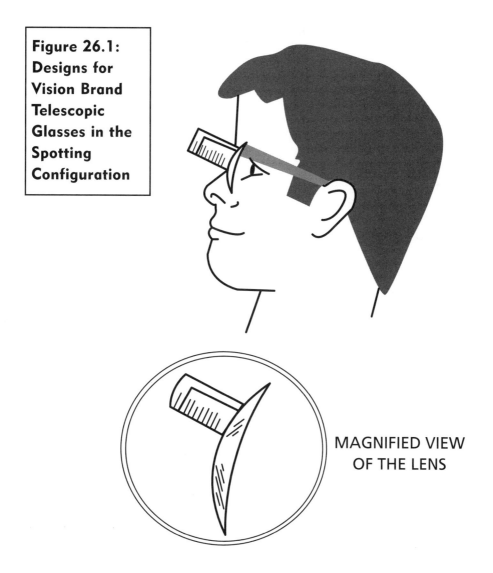

Figure 26.1: Designs for Vision Brand Telescopic Glasses in the Spotting Configuration

MAGNIFIED VIEW
OF THE LENS

See Part V for more discussion about driving with telescopic glasses.

CHAPTER 27

Aids for Watching Television

Disease	Usefulness (scale 1–10)	See note number
Cataracts	8–9–10	N/A
Diabetic retinopathy	10	N/A
Glaucoma	1–2–3	1
Macular degeneration	10	N/A
Retinitis pigmentosa	1–2–3	1

Scale

1 =   Offers little if any help for someone with this disease.

4–5–6 = Moderately effective for someone with this disease.

10 =   Very effective for someone with this disease.

(Other ratings can be gauged accordingly.)

Note

1. Aids in this chapter are of little help to persons who have experienced severe field loss.

Get Closer

Television has become our primary source of news and information. Those who can't see it miss a lot. Unlike what our parents told us as youngsters (or what we told our own children), getting closer to the set solves this problem. Sit two feet from the screen and use eccentric viewing, if it is appropriate. If you have macular problems, don't look at the center of the screen. Fixate on the cabinet around the screen. You will see the screen as well as a person with normal vision sees it from twenty feet away.

Getting closer is sometimes a problem. Large console models may be too low to the ground. They can be raised to eye level by using concrete blocks. Paint the blocks an appropriate color to minimize a spouse's objections, or splurge a little and have a professional carpenter build an attractive stand for this purpose. Table-model TVs can be placed on the edge of a table where the patient can get close.

The large-screen, rear-projection TVs are great. I have a forty-six-inch Sony I view from six feet; I see it fine without other aids. Naturally, since I have macular problems, I must also use eccentric viewing. These models cost $1,500 to $2,500. Use caution when shopping for rear-projection TVs. Compare brands before buying. Many have a very narrow viewing angle. Picture quality drops dramatically when they are viewed from a little to the side rather than straight on. Rear-projection TVs do not work well in brightly lighted rooms, and they must be viewed from eye level. The viewer's head should be level with the center of the screen.

Using Telescopic Aids

Special telescopic aids allow the visually impaired to sit back in a favorite easy chair and still see the screen. The user can't read the credits after a movie, but she can see the program quite well. One Sunday afternoon, I demonstrated one of these aids to an elderly doctor. He was a football fan, and the Cowboys were playing. He settled into his recliner and took the aid. He slipped it on and then sat up, excitedly waving his arms. "I can see their eyebrows!" This brief story sufficiently proves the point.

Many low-vision specialists are not impressed with the value of this type of aid for television. On the other hand, I have sold hundreds of this type of aid. The difference was that I was in the patients' homes, where they could try the aid while viewing their own set.

The same telescopes used for driving can be mounted in glasses pointing straight ahead in the constant-use configuration. They work very well for viewing movies, stage plays, opera, and TV, as well as for many other visual tasks. The 4X Expanded Field prismatic scopes made by Designs for Vision are best for this type of viewing. The 2.2X Galilean scope is much lighter and cheaper, if its power is sufficient. Depending on the power and type of scope, these cost from $500 to $2,500.

A pair of 4X prismatic scopes as mentioned above weighs about 3.6 ounces. This is very heavy. It takes a long time to adjust to carrying this much weight on the nose. When you first begin using them, take them off at every commercial. After about a year, you should be able to wear them through a complete TV movie without removing them.

Beecher Research Company offers an excellent aid that is less expensive than the Designs for Vision glasses. It is a pair of binoculars in spectacle frames. The ones I tried were 7X. They have a fairly comfortable strap to help hold them on the head. The nose pads are a new design, so although the glasses weigh three ounces, they seem much lighter. They cost about $275 when ordered direct from Beecher. Their field of view is not as wide as the Designs for Vision 4X prismatic scopes, but the lower cost compensates for this. Many people will need help from a professional in properly adjusting these sport glasses, even though directions are supplied. The Beecher address is in Appendix B.

Selsi also offers a fine TV aid. Their model 227 with glass lenses is simply a 2.5X pair of binoculars in spectacle frames. The glasses are heavy, weighing about 2.7 ounces. Use the procedure described above to develop tolerance for this weight. The Selsi model 227 costs about $85 and is available by prescription from the New York Lighthouse for the Blind, Optical Aids Service. One size fits all. If a patient wants to avoid the hassle of getting a prescription, they are also available from Bossert Specialties for about $138. See Appendix B for contact information.

Selsi also offers model 229 Sport Glasses in 2.8X with plastic lenses. They are lighter and acceptable, but the optical quality is not as good as that provided by the 227. Obtain them from the New York Lighthouse with a prescription for $39, or from Bossert Specialties without a prescription for $95.

Another brand is the Eschenbach 3X Sport Glasses. They are much lighter than the glasses listed above, but more expensive than the Selsi, and their field of view is narrower. They list for $134 with a prescription from the New York Lighthouse. Bossert Specialties sells them without a prescription for about $200.

The Eschenbach and Selsi Sport Glasses have an adjustment for pupillary distance (PD). PD is the distance between the two pupils. The scopes move in or out to center them directly in front of the pupils. Ask a doctor for help if you have trouble adjusting them correctly.

Some people may question the use of 2.5X and 3X scopes for a person who needs 10X to see 20/20. This is a legitimate question, and the answer is that although someone may need a visual acuity of 20/20 to read, 20/20 vision is not required to see and enjoy TV.

CHAPTER 28

Aids for Writing

When people lose vision, they also lose handwriting ability. For about a year after losing vision, one's hand will continue to shape the letters well enough to be readable. But over time, when a person can't see to shape letters, the hand "forgets" how to do it and handwriting deteriorates.

Research conducted by the Veteran's Administration proved that the best writing aid is the video visual aid discussed in Chapter 22. It allows the user to sit comfortably and shape letters properly by watching the screen.

Some of the visually impaired can write with reading glasses, but the glasses' very short focal length makes it difficult to get a pen between the lens and the paper. A better choice is a separate pair of glasses about one-half the power of reading glasses. Handwritten material is larger than print, so the patient can use less power. The one-half power will double the focal distance, allowing more space between the lens and the paper. Even with half-power lenses, it is necessary to bend forward until the eye is about three inches above the paper. This is uncomfortable, and some people simply can't do it. Those who cannot assume this awkward bending position should use a clipboard. Hold the clipboard close to the eye without bending the torso. Another alternative is to use a raised, slanted stand on top of the desk to bring the paper to eye level, minimizing how much one must bend to write.

Felt-tip pens are another very helpful writing aid. The broad lines they produce are more visible than the lines from standard pens. They are available from office-supply stores in a variety of colors. For most visually impaired users, a medium point in black is best.

Telephone directories are a pain. Create your own personal directory of frequently called numbers using a felt-tip pen. Print phone numbers in a spiral notebook; make the numbers one-half inch to one inch tall. If you get close and use eccentric viewing (if appropriate), you can read the entries without other aids.

Don't forget to use wide-line paper as well, described in Chapter 20.

CHAPTER 29

Handling Money

Persons with visual impairment sometimes hold out a handful of change to store clerks and tell them, "Take what you need." This is not recommended! Too many people will do exactly that!

Coins are more difficult to manage than paper currency. Quarters have a milled edge, while nickels do not. Pennies are darker in color than dimes. These observations help, but it often takes too much time to find exact change when others are waiting in line.

For the most part, I solve this problem by avoiding it. I pay for purchases using bills and put the change in my pocket. Back home, I toss the change into a bowl. When the bowl is full, I use magnifying spectacles to sort and roll the coins for deposit in the bank. Nowadays, many banks will sort and roll coins for their customers. They have coin-sorting machines, so the task is quick and easy for them. These are simple solutions to the problem.

Paper currency is another matter. Electronic gadgets help the blind identify the denomination of bills. These are for use by totally blind persons and are rarely used by the partially sighted. The totally blind use another technique to keep money straight. They tear one corner off a five-dollar bill, two corners off a ten, etc. Federal officials frown on this practice, but no one will fault the totally blind for doing it.

There are several ways to identify paper money. I use the following system. I've compartmentalized my wallet. One-dollar and five-dollar bills are kept in the main part of the wallet. The ones and fives are separated from each other by a card of some kind. Ten-dollar bills are kept with the fives, but always on the inside of the fives, near the card. Twenty-dollar bills, folded in half with the "green" side out, are placed in a separate compartment beneath credit cards. Fifties, folded in half with the "blue" side out, are in another compartment.

This procedure helps, but it does not prevent occasional mistakes. I once gave away a fifty when I thought I was handing over a twenty. A friend gave away a hundred-dollar bill, thinking it was a one. It is not surprising that the visually impaired make these mistakes or that people take advantage of them.

Minimize mistakes by using residual vision! Do not trust any system completely. Before handing over a twenty from the twenty-dollar-bill compartment in your wallet or purse, bring it up close and look at it. To assist in this process, I personally avoid use of hundred-dollar bills. I also avoid tens whenever possible, because while my compartmentalized-wallet method provides a system for dealing with tens, having a third type of bill in the same compartment increases the probability of mistakes.

If you use the first basic principle of "getting closer" (within two or three inches), you will make fewer mistakes. To avoid making any errors, take the time to use a favorite low-vision aid to read each bill.

CHAPTER 30

Playing Cards (and Analyzing Visual Tasks)

This chapter provides information on how to play card games. The primary purpose of this information is to offer an example of how to analyze visual tasks related to any activity. Analyzing a task is the first step in selecting an aid for help in performing it.

Visual tasks are defined by the distance between the visual target and the eye. Card games differ, but generally, a player must be able to see the cards held in the hand and those played in the center of the table. Stud poker requires seeing across the table. In bridge there are three visual tasks: watching the hand, the table center, and the dummy across the table.

The multiple visual tasks involved in playing bridge create a low-vision-specialist's nightmare, because so many different distances are involved. Lenses are not like the human eye. They are not adaptable. Each lens has its own focal length. To play bridge, the player would need three different tools, to focus at three different distances. The play in poker is slow enough that one might use a Selsi or Walters Near Focus Monocular that will focus at all distances required. When playing bridge, however, things move much faster, and there isn't enough time to play it comfortably with only one aid. In this case, having three different aids wouldn't help either.

Telescopic glasses with two telescopes focused at different distances are a possibility. For example, read the dummy hand with the left eye through one telescope and read cards in the center of the table with the right eye though another telescope. A person could read cards in the hand with magnifying bifocals added to the carrier lenses below the scopes. Such a pair of glasses would be quite expensive, very heavy, and impractical in my opinion.

There are other ways to approach this visual task. There are two kinds of playing cards: regular (bridge) and jumbo indexed. A person who is visually impaired can read either of these in his hand with magnifying glasses.

Special cards for people with low vision also exist. They are printed with super-large numbers, and my favorite brand is color-coded. Spades and hearts are black and red, as usual. But clubs are blue and diamonds are green. Players with visual impairment can manage with these low-vision playing cards simply by bending over and getting closer. I play bridge once a month using these cards. Friends recognize my special need and accept use of the cards.

A floor lamp beside the table will also help. In bridge, the dummy hand normally stays on the opposite side of the table — but it does not have to. Pull it over until it is close enough for you to bend forward and see the cards. Spread the cards out so they do not overlap. This helps as much as additional light.

I built a board to hold my cards without overlapping, and getting close to them is easy. The board is one-eighth-inch plywood and very light. It holds five cards across and has rows to hold four suits. A piece of molding creates shelves for each suit. Having the special low-vision cards fully exposed without overlapping, I can view them easily without a low-vision aid. I also use the combined techniques of eccentric viewing and getting closer. These boards are not available commercially, but perhaps you can make your own. A local cabinetmaker could also build one.

Using low-vision playing cards and employing some ingenuity allow many persons with visual impairment to play card games without additional help. If more help is needed, ask your fellow players to speak what they play. Remember that trying to be too independent may handicap you as much as your visual disability.

When it comes to performing a given task, study it carefully. Think logically about the factors involved. The important variable is: how far away is the visual target? This will dictate the type of aid or skill needed. Don't be afraid to try something new. Optical aids are not the only choice. Search for and find new ways of doing things that persons with normal vision do.

About two years ago, I began making knives. There is no way I can see well enough to hold a piece of steel and grind it into shape. That requires good vision. Getting close enough to the belt sander to use reading glasses wasn't a good solution either. I learned the hard way that steel sparks pit glass lenses! Sparks bounce off plastic lenses, but they burn into glass, ruining the lenses.

It took me ten years to devise a way to make knives, but the idea finally came. I designed and made a jig that allows me to grind blades without good vision. Necessity is the mother of invention, they say. When conventional aids do not serve your needs, don't be afraid to try something new.

CHAPTER 31

Reading a Watch

Keeping track of time is not as hard for the visually impaired as some might imagine. It is simple to take out a magnifier and read one's watch, but many people prefer not to do this.

This book has already discussed large-print appliances and "talking" products. Both large-print and talking clocks and watches are available through the recommended catalogs. The watches announce the time when a button is pressed, and most are quite affordable (less than $50). However, the use of talking watches in church or other public gatherings is distracting to others.

I prefer a more expensive watch and one that does not talk. I find that the size of the numbers on the dial is less important than the width of the hands. If the hands are wide and bold, you can tell time by the position of the hands, without reading the numbers.

Look for a watch with a black face and white, bold hands. A second hand is acceptable, but visually impaired persons occasionally see it instead of the minute and hour hands. A watch repairman can remove the second hand if it gives trouble.

Look for a large watch, one with an uncluttered dial. Extra gadgets on the face such as tachometers and stop-watch dials are distracting and make the watch hard to read. Avoid watches with gold faces and gold hands. Avoid all watches with narrow hands.

I have owned two diver's watches, a Bulova and a Seiko. They are waterproof down to ridiculous depths, but more importantly, they have clear, easily seen dials. By lifting them to within a few inches of the eye, one can easily read them.

CHAPTER 32

A Survival Kit

A person with normal vision would never leave home without her eyeballs. Since the low-vision aids used by the person with subnormal vision are in a sense her eyeballs, she should never leave home without them. She should always carry them in a pocket or purse.

I worked for many years traveling throughout three large states. There was no one around to read a road map for me. I had no help reading menus. I was forced to operate independently. The method I devised to meet this challenge might interest some readers.

I designed and made a case to carry all my aids. At a craft store, I purchased a box measuring ten inches by fourteen inches by three inches deep. Inside, using one-eighth-inch balsa wood covered with plastic cloth, I fashioned compartments for the aids I needed at the time. I covered the box's exterior in black leather and added a handle. In the case, I carried the following:

FOR WRITING:

◆ Half-eye glasses: +12 D.

FOR READING:

◆ Half-eye glasses: +18 D.

◆ Half-eye glasses: +24 D.

FOR READING CITY AND ROAD MAPS:

◆ Stand magnifier: Sloan Focusable, +53 D. (This aid is no longer available.)

FOR DISTANCE VIEWING:

◆ Selsi model 164, 8X20 near-focus monocular

◆ 6X telescopic glasses, one telescope in spotting configuration (for driving)

◆ 4X telescopic glasses, two scopes mounted in constant use configuration (for movies)

As my vision became worse, I dropped the weaker reading glasses and added half-eye spectacles in +36 D. and a pair of Corning light-amber sunglasses. I always carried a +20 D. pocket magnifier in a pocket and a backup pair of driving glasses in another case.

This was my survival kit. With it, I could operate independently.

I include this information for two reasons. Other persons who are visually impaired may have the same need to operate independently, without assistance of any kind. A kit such as this will help achieve this objective.

I also wish to illustrate that no single aid is sufficient for independence. Every person with visual impairment must own a battery of aids for both near and distance viewing.

Yesterday I received a call from a lady who read my book on macular degeneration a year ago. She had gone to a low-vision specialist. He fitted her with reading glasses. Since the disease was just beginning at the time, he fitted her with rather weak lenses. At first she could read with the glasses, but her visual acuity dropped, and now she can no longer read with them. For several months, she has been unable to read. She didn't know her doctor could provide stronger aids.

Progressive deterioration is the pattern for most diseases. Over time, the conditions become more severe. **It is not a waste of money to buy glasses that work today but will not work a year from now.** I have never bought a pair of glasses that fully lost their usefulness, even though I needed to replace them with stronger ones. For example, my writing glasses today were yesteryear's reading glasses. Remember, although it is unlikely you will ever need lenses so strong, reading lenses are available up to +100 D.

Part V

Specialized Knowledge
and Skills

CHAPTER 33

Education

Educating the visually impaired requires special knowledge and skills. As a rule, regular teachers do not possess this expertise. Only teachers certified to teach the visually impaired receive this training.

Some school districts have special classes for the visually impaired, but many districts "mainstream" these students, so that the visually impaired attend the same classes as students with normal vision. In these cases, specially trained teachers advise and help the regular teachers.

Many schools offer special equipment, like video visual aids, for student use. Even small school districts have on staff a consultant for the visually impaired, hired by the state education agency. This person works with several schools and teachers or assists regular teachers in the education of the visually impaired.

Recordings for the Blind

The organization Recordings for the Blind (see Appendix B) provides an invaluable service for the blind and visually impaired. They maintain a library of textbooks and resource books in recorded form for scholars from grade four through the doctoral level. They also supply books and professional journals for persons who have completed their formal education but who need to continue reading in their field. They offer other materials as well, such as recorded Boy Scout merit-badge books. During my doctoral program, I obtained half of the books I needed from this organization.

The books come to the user through the U.S. Postal Service as Free Matter for the Blind, and they can be returned the same way. (See Chapter 7, "Perks and Privileges," for more about this program which allows the visually impaired to send material through the mail postage-free.) The student may keep the books for the entire duration of the course.

If a book or a new edition of a book is not available, Recordings for the Blind will record it. As it is being recorded, they send it out chapter by chapter. They use what is called the Library of Congress format in recording these books. The playing speed is $^{15}/_{16}$ inches per second (ips) in a four-track format. A machine provided by the Library of Congress's Talking Book Program will play these special recordings. Although music must be recorded at faster speeds, $^{15}/_{16}$ ips is sufficient for spoken material. Before purchasing a recorder, make sure it will play the Library of Congress format, that is, four tracks per tape at $^{15}/_{16}$ ips. You will not find machines with this capability at electronics stores. Check the catalogs I recommended.

The sound quality of these tapes is excellent, and professionals in the applicable fields generally do the reading. If the book is a psychology book, a psychologist reads it. If it is a math book, a mathematician reads it. This practice ensures that names of people in the field and technical terms are pronounced properly.

Educational Goals

Educators talk about a "body of knowledge." They have identified skills and knowledge they believe are essential for all students to learn before high school graduation. Students must learn the body of knowledge assigned to their grade level.

Many states administer achievement tests to students each

year to determine whether the teachers have done their job. Test scores provide information on how well the students have learned, but also give a measure of the success or failure of the teachers. Little wonder educators become preoccupied with this body of knowledge!

Many psychologists have criticized Sigmund Freud, the father of psychology, for inadequately estimating the impact of societal forces on the development of personality. Eric Erickson, one of his students, made this observation long ago. Erickson pursued his belief that society was a strong molder of personality, and he studied indigenous societies in an attempt to identify variables common to all. What he learned is worthy of attention.

1. He found that each culture had its own unique survival tool. For the Eskimos, it was a spear. For the plains Indians of North America, it was the bow and arrow. For the African pygmy, it was the blowgun.

2. Erickson observed that both a man's status in his community and his wealth were related to his skill in the use of the survival tool. The most skilled in the tribe earned the most respect. They were also the wealthiest. They fed their families well. Those not skillful with the tool often went hungry, and they held less important positions in the tribe.

3. In each society Erickson studied, the parents gave this basic survival tool in toy form to their male children when they were about four years of age.

What about our society? What is our basic survival tool? The answer is so simple and obvious it eludes most people.

The basic survival tool in Western society is the pen. The pen, of course, represents reading and writing skills. The best-paid people and those who hold the highest positions of respect in Western society are persons who excel in these skills. As in indigenous cultures, people in our society give the basic survival tool to children when they are about four. Most children are not given pens or pencils, but they are given the toy equivalents. They are given chalkboards and chalk. They are given coloring books and crayons. Intuitively, people know that children need to begin learning the coordination needed for writing, even if they do not think of the pen as a survival tool.

Research has proven that the one variable most closely related to success in school is the I.Q. of the student. Almost all I.Q. tests are a test of vocabulary. They are reading tests!

I agree with educators that there exists a body of knowledge each student should acquire. Reading is just one of the skills incorporated in that body of knowledge, but I assert the following: reading must be the **primary** objective in educating the visually impaired. For the visually impaired, the overall body of knowledge must always take a back seat to reading skill. Omit geography if necessary. Skip over government and history, but teach the visually impaired to read! Expand their vocabulary. This should be uppermost in teachers' minds when they work with the visually impaired. If parents want to promote the education of a child with visual impairment, they should constantly remind public-school teachers of this objective. With reading ability, the student can acquire on his or her own the unique body of knowledge he or she needs. The inability to read well means menial jobs and never acquiring the rest of the body of knowledge.

Why is promoting this skill especially important for the visually impaired? Isn't it true that all students — the normally sighted **and** the visually impaired — can obtain the rest of the body of knowledge only if they become good readers? Yes, but the visually impaired have a special incentive for becoming superior and practiced readers. Review Chapter 3, "How We See." Humans **learn** to see, and reading is a function of memory. The brain must learn to identify coded electronic signals from the eye for each word in the student's vocabulary. The student memorizes the code by seeing it repeatedly. The student must reinforce the memory of that code for the rest of his or her life, much the same way Tiger Woods must reinforce and perfect his muscles' "memory" of the perfect golf swing. The way Tiger does this is to practice his swing countless times every day. The way the student reinforces his or her memory of the codes that represent words is to see them continually.

For the normally sighted in our society, reading remains automatic, because all day long, every day, they encounter written material designed for their eyes to see. By contrast, the visually impaired must make a conscious effort to seek out reading material that their eyes can see, or to employ visual aids and techniques that enable them to read written material designed for those with normal vision. Therefore, it is tempting for someone with subnormal vision to avoid making the extra effort required to read. So, all other educational objectives must be secondary to reading.

Attending College

College students with visual impairment receive less direct assistance than students in the public schools; however, help is available. Universities that receive federal funds are required to assign someone to assist handicapped students. This person will not read for the visually impaired, but he can arrange special testing situations and help with preregistration and similar matters. Find out who this advocate for handicapped students is on your campus.

Students with visual impairment who go through the public school system learn skills and techniques that continue to be productive in college, but college work requires additional skills. The following sections contain information on how to function in the college classroom, how to record lecture notes, how to use recorded books, how to hire readers, and how to take tests if one can neither read nor write. Some of the material will be of value to public school students as well.

It may appear in some cases that I am advocating blind rehabilitation instead of vision rehabilitation. That is not so. This book emphasizes reading for oneself, but the quantity of material to be read in college dictates use of other technologies. For example, the visually impaired rarely read faster than 100 words per minute (wpm), perhaps 150 wpm with a video visual aid. Some professors assert that a person can't keep up in college reading this slowly. I tend to agree, but I also know that motivation can negate slow reading speeds. With recorded material, one can use compressed speech or speed-hearing and triple one's reading speed. The efficiency of this technology dictates its use.

Taking Notes

All college students must be able to take notes on lectures they attend, and they must be able to read the blackboard.

In 1973, I visited a rehab center for the blind as a part of my doctoral internship. An instructor in charge of college preparation was teaching a client who was totally blind to write so the client could take notes in class. The instructor's solution was impractical. Who would read the notes for the blind student? What good would his notes be to him?

In the early stages of vision impairment, students may still be able to take notes and read them later. Those who have this ability should use it. But most students with subnormal vision will need additional help to supplement their limited note-taking ability. Deal with this task by using tape recorders, but learn to use them correctly.

Never record an entire lecture. In some classes, teachers forbid it. I've met professors who did not permit recorders in their class-rooms. Assure professors that the recorder is for dictating notes only. If they still will not permit use of the recorder, consult the department head, or better still, the school's advocate for handi-capped students.

When preparing for tests, there isn't enough time to listen to complete lecture recordings. It takes too long, and it is tedious to listen to the same lecture repeatedly. Other students write notes during a lecture, outlining what the professor says. Instead of writing notes, the visually impaired dictate them into a recorder.

Careful selection of the equipment used facilitates note taking. If possible, use a recorder that has an On/Off switch on the micro-phone. Put the machine in record mode, then turn it off and on at the mike as needed. Do not let it run all the time. Machines without a switch on the mike will work, but they are less efficient.

Hold the microphone close, touching the lips. Most recorders today have an automatic volume control while in recording mode. Whisper notes into the microphone. This will not disturb other students, so there is no need to sit in the back of the classroom. The whispered comments come through loud and clear when the recording is played back.

Use two machines if possible. One should be a portable, battery-operated unit that is small enough to carry easily. Beware of very small recorders that lack needed features or ones that use cassettes too small to be practical. A Talking Book Machine furnished by the Library of Congress is a backup system only. It should not be one of the basic units since it will not record. It is a playback machine only.

Keep a second, larger recorder at home. Both the larger machine and the portable one must have jacks available so they can be connected to each other by cable. Copy material from one to the other. The ability to copy data recorded on the portable machine to the larger machine is essential. Copying from the larger to the portable machine may prove helpful at times, but copying from the portable to the larger is essential.

The larger machine must be able to play four-track tapes recorded at $^{15}/_{16}$ inches per second (ips). A portable recorder that will do the same is a convenience. The portable unit need not include a variable speed control (or compressed speech; see below), but the larger unit must have one or the other. "Variable speed" does not mean that it has several recording and playback speeds. It means that any recording speed can be sped up or slowed down.

Use separate cassette tapes to dictate notes for each class. Upon arrival at home, copy the lecture notes to the larger recorder on a master tape dedicated to each course.

It is a good idea to begin each class session by dictating the course title and the day and date of that recording. Example: "History 101, Wednesday, September 17." Erase this identifying material when copying it to the master tape at home.

When copying data from one tape to another, it is unnecessary to run the machine at the speed at which it was recorded. Save time by doubling or tripling the speed. For example, consider a recording made at $^{15}/_{16}$ ips. If the portable machine has a set speed, double this ($1^{7}/_{8}$ ips). Then set both machines on $1^{7}/_{8}$ and start copying. When played back at the original recorded speed, it will sound fine.

Other students read their notes. The visually impaired listen to theirs. Fifty-minute lectures compressed into ten-minute outlines make it easy to review notes. The student using tape recorders will appreciate the condensed form of these notes when the time comes to prepare for a test. Imagine the time it would take to review full recordings of all lectures attended.

Be sure to master the skills of using the recorders and making copies before getting to college. Learn these skills during the summer before the first semester in school. As noted earlier in this book, you will not find recorders that play four-track tapes at $15/16$ of an inch per second at an electronics store. You can find them in the low-vision aids catalogs I recommend.

Recorded class notes in outline form save time, but one must also read the textbook. There are ways to reduce listening time. While working on my doctorate, from 1969–1973, I used variable-speed tape recorders. These machines had set running speeds of $1^7/_8$, $3^3/_4$ ips, and $7^1/_2$ ips, controlled by three sizes of drive pulleys. They also had variable-speed motors. Any playback speed would run slower or faster than the recorded speed. Class notes could be recorded at a given speed and then listened to at a faster speed. Increasing the speed of the tape moved it through the machine faster, reducing listening time.

Playing a tape faster than its recorded speed produces Donald Duck gibberish. But if the speed is gradually increased, one can learn to understand this gibberish. Friends with normal vision will not be able to understand this gibberish. They will spread myths about their friend who has developed amazing powers because of his blindness! (The totally blind have lived with these myths for generations.) This skill really isn't difficult to learn. Gradually increase the listening speed. Even the normally sighted can hear faster than they think they can.

Speed-hearing requires greater concentration than regular listening. I found that my residual vision was a hindrance. As I listened to tapes, my eyes picked up objects in the room and my mind wandered off the subject. Shutting my eyes to block out visual stimuli helped, but when I did so, I went to sleep. I solved the problem by finding a pair of sunglasses with large lenses and painting the lenses with opaque fingernail polish. When I wore the glasses my eyes remained open, but visual stimuli were blocked.

Persons using so much recorded material need comfortable earphones. Avoid the "bugs" that fit in the ear. Get earphones that cover both ears. They will help blot out other sounds and aid concentration.

This is off the subject of vision, but my posterior got tired sitting and listening to tapes. But if I lay down, I fell asleep. A lounge-type lawn chair allowed me to sit up with my legs supported by the footrest. I was more comfortable and remained alert.

About the time I graduated, in 1973, a new product called "compressed speech" was introduced. It has greatly increased reading efficiency for the visually impaired. The psychologist who researched compressed speech cut recording tape into quarter-inch lengths. He then patched it back together in the proper order, leaving out every fourth piece on some tapes, every third piece on other tapes, and so on. Even though he'd discarded parts of the tape, the result was still understandable to experimental subjects when run through a recorder at standard speed. Oral reading is about 150 words per minute. The researcher learned that students with normal vision could speed up their hearing to about 475 wpm.

The next step was the development of machines that would do this clipping electronically. These machines have variable-speed motors. As the speed increases, the machines electronically clip out material so the tape goes through the machine faster. The machines emit a clipping sound as the tape plays, but there is no Donald Duck gibberish.

Many people believe that the blind develop superior hearing. They do not. They simply learn to use what all humans have. The person who has vision doesn't need to hone these skills, but the blind do so easily and naturally. The person with partial vision finds himself somewhere between these two groups, canted toward the normally sighted. As long as there is vision, people use it. Nonetheless, with conscious effort, the partially sighted can develop the ability to listen to tapes faster than they were recorded. The compressed-speech machines are better and are preferable, but even the Donald Duck gibberish is understandable with practice. For example, I recorded tapes at $1^7/_8$ ips and played them back at $3^3/_4$ ips. This cut my reading time in half, or gave me the ability to read 300 wpm. With compressed-speech machines, listening speed increases to between 400 and 500 wpm.

Recorders used by students receive heavy use and need regular maintenance. Give them this maintenance and they perform well, but without it, sound quality drops dramatically. Between semesters, always perform the following maintenance on recorders.

1. Magnetic recording tape is made of iron oxide on a plastic ribbon. The iron oxide rubs off on the recorder's playback and recording heads. It will build up on the heads and create background noise and poor sound quality. Learn how to remove the case from the recorder to expose the recording heads. Use a cotton swab dampened with alcohol (not dripping wet) to clean these shiny surfaces. Wood alcohol or special head-cleaner works best, but rubbing alcohol can also be used.

2. The tape passing by the heads and tape guides causes them to become magnetized. This interferes with sound quality. Demagnetize the heads with a special product called a head demagnetizer, available at electronics stores. Follow the directions carefully. Do not wear a watch while doing the task, and keep all tapes and computer disks away from the work area. Head demagnetizers destroy data on recording tapes and computer disks.

3. Most recorders use rubber belts in the drive mechanism. Carefully clean the belts with alcohol, and remove oil from the pulley grooves they run in. Carefully oil the pulley shafts with light machine oil, available at hardware stores and some supermarkets.

Blackboards

Blackboards gave me fits until I discovered low-vision aids halfway through my doctoral program. They were the primary reason I began a search for help. Some professors were more cooperative than others, and some were totally inept at helping to meet my needs around this issue.

I used several methods to deal with blackboards.

1. Some professors speak aloud as they write on the blackboard. If they do, the visually impaired can manage without seeing what is written. If a professor does not speak as he writes, ask for verbal stimuli. Most will comply and speak aloud when they know there is a person with vision loss in the class.

2. I had professors who seemed unable to do this. I asked them to speak what they were writing, and they complied for a few words, then slipped back into silence. After this

happened a few times with one professor, I got out of my seat and walked to the blackboard. I stood close behind the professor where I could see the blackboard. The professor didn't like it. His space had been invaded.

3. In 1971, I learned about low-vision aids and found a simple solution to my blackboard-reading problem. I used a telescope (monocular) to read the blackboard. Many telescopes will not focus on targets inside a given distance. This depends on the power and type of telescope, but with some scopes there is a limit to how close one can be to the target. Sit close to the board, but not so close that the telescope will not focus. Telescopes with near-focus capability avoid this problem, for example, the Selsi 8X20, model 164.

Handheld telescopes in binocular or monocular form are available in powers from 2X to about 20X. The more powerful they are, the larger they are. Sometimes one must compromise between visual ability and a practical size.

Eye-care professionals are keenly aware of research proving that persons with normal vision cannot use very powerful handheld telescopes. As the power increases, hand movement dramatically reduces visual acuity. This is true for the visually impaired as well, but they can tolerate more movement than the normally sighted can. (I have met excellent low-vision specialists who were unaware of this fact.) Why the visually impaired can tolerate more hand movement when holding a handheld telescope remains unclear, but it may relate to the fact that their brains are accustomed to processing weak or distorted signals from the eyes. The visually impaired can handle using a powerful scope, hand movement and all, even if the visual ability of the normally sighted would be destroyed under such circumstances.

How strong should the scope be? Selsi, Walters, and many other manufacturers produce miniature scopes in powers up to 10X. Both binoculars and monoculars are available. Monoculars are for one eye. One-eye scopes work well, and they are lighter, less bulky, and easier to carry. They fit easily into a pocket or purse. Recall that a 10X scope gives 20/20 vision to a person with a visual acuity of 20/200, and rarely will reading a blackboard require vision as good as 20/20. Those who need even more power can obtain it. Scopes in 20X are available that are about a foot long. Carry these on shoulder straps.

Designs for Vision (see Appendix B) produces prescription telescopic glasses that are available in powers from 1.7 to 10. I completed the last two years of my doctoral work wearing a pair of these in 2.2X. Often they were not strong enough to read the blackboard, so I carried a small handheld 2.5X monocular. When necessary, I used both at the same time by holding the handheld scope in front of the scope mounted in the glasses.

Using Recorded Books

A few more words about ordering books from Recordings for the Blind may prove helpful. Recordings for the Blind requires one month to fill orders, even when they have the books recorded and ready to ship. Therefore, you need to place orders a month before the semester begins.

While one semester is in progress, the university is planning the next. They are deciding what courses to offer and who will teach them and in what classroom. Weeks before a new semester begins, someone will have this information. Department heads are the best source. Try to work out next semester's schedule before the end of the present term. Once you've done this, go to the professors who will teach the courses and ask what textbooks they plan to use. Most, but not all, will know and provide this information. Try to place your order for recorded books a month in advance.

Using Readers

Fifty percent of my textbooks came from Recordings for the Blind, but I was unwilling to wait for them to record books they did not already have in stock. I had the remaining ones recorded personally, using a reader service provided at the expense of the Veteran's Administration.

Clients of the VA, the commission for the blind, or visual services usually are provided funds to hire readers. In some cases, the agencies provide a video visual aid. This, in my opinion, saves them money, but students who are visually impaired will need reader service as well. This is true especially when doing research in the library. Reading a card catalog with low-vision aids is difficult, and finding a specific book on the shelves is even harder. Many universities have computerized catalogs, but they do not have computers equipped with large-print displays. These limitations make it almost mandatory to have access to reader service.

Magnifying glasses and even handheld magnifiers work on computer screens. Try them to see if they will work for you. Those who use stand magnifiers can put the base against the eye and lean very close to the screen until it is in focus. Most near-focus monoculars (like the Selsi 8X20, model 164) allow users to read computer screens. Adjust them to their nearest focal point, and then move close until the screen is in focus.

My experience using readers may be of help.

1. Do not depend on volunteer students if it can be avoided. When needed most, they are busy preparing for their own

tests. **Hire** readers whenever possible. The rate of pay for a reader is about the same as the minimum wages paid by the university to student employees in the dining halls.

2. Do not hire persons to read who can only work in their own homes. I tried this at first, and time after time I was let down. Too often, the material wasn't ready when I needed it. After taking a test without having read the material and scoring a thirty on it, I changed procedures. Meet readers at a designated place on a scheduled basis. My readers reported to my home and worked from 1:00 P.M. to 5:00 P.M. each weekday afternoon.

   Finding a suitable place to meet readers can be tricky. If the reader cannot come to your room or residence, ask permission to use a room in the student union or some other campus building.

3. A spouse can provide reading assistance, but do not use him or her as a primary source. Family members may not have adequate time to devote to this activity, even though they would like to help.

4. Finding a reader is not difficult if you pay them. Announce in class that a job is available for someone to work as a reader. Another possibility is to place "Help Wanted" notices in dorm elevators. When ending their employment, my readers were extremely helpful in finding a replacement. They knew other persons who wanted a job.

5. Do not hire someone simply because he or she is interested. Test applicants first. Oral reading ability varies greatly, and some voices are more understandable than others, especially when using speed-hearing or compressed speech. Record

each applicant reading a passage. Time the applicants to calculate the number of words read per minute. Send them home, then listen to each tape. Compare readers before hiring. Some voices allow faster reading than others.

6. Many fraternities and sororities contribute time to the blind as readers. This may work better than depending on one volunteer, because another member of the club may fill in when the regular reader is busy. Depending on volunteers is risky, however. A paid employee is more reliable.

7. Never sit listening to a reader read. Always have them record the material, then listen to the tape later at a faster speed. If it becomes necessary to listen to the reader personally, record the material while listening. After the reader is gone, the material will still be available on tape.

8. Most recorders with a remote microphone will have a cord long enough to hang the mike around the reader's neck. Point the mike up, and it will produce better recordings than putting the mike on a table beside the reader.

Preparing for Tests

My first semester as a doctoral student was the spring of 1969. I took three undergraduate courses and one doctoral-level course. At the time, I could still read, although doing so was slow and painfully inefficient. Since I could still manage it, however inefficiently, I used my reading ability and avoided the onerous task of learning to learn by hearing. I did all right that semester, scoring two A's and two B's, but it became clear a change was needed.

When the summer term came, I decided to develop new skills. I selected a course in psychological testing. The first day of class was a Monday morning. The professor told the students what to expect. The class would have a long, multiple-choice test on each of the next four Mondays. The last Monday would be the final exam.

Determined to learn by hearing alone, I studied for the first test by listening repeatedly to the recorded text. The test was to cover five long, technical chapters. Often bored, I went to sleep while listening to the same chapter the fourth or fifth time.

The following Monday, with fear and trepidation, I took the test. There were twelve doctoral students in the class, and my score was the fourth highest. No one in the class scored better than the high eighties.

The second test covered even more material. I hadn't enough time to listen to all the material five or six times. I took notes while reading several chapters, and I listened to others repeatedly. I scored third highest on the second test, and again, no one in the class broke the ninety-point barrier.

For the third test, I still emphasized listening to the tapes, but I also took a few more notes. I scored second highest in the class, and again no one broke ninety. For the fourth test, my study pattern remained about the same, and my results the same. I scored second highest, and no one broke ninety.

A week later was the final exam. It covered far too much material to consider listening to the whole book again. I spent a little time looking over the notes I had made, then I went in to take the test. I scored ninety-four, the top grade in the class and the only score to break the ninety barrier.

Here I must confess that I "cheated." I didn't use hidden notes or anything like that. I simply studied the tests given by this professor. I analyzed the four tests we'd already taken and found that the professor favored the "D" response 50 percent of the time.

With four responses per question, this percentage should have been 25. When I took the final exam, if I didn't have a clue to the correct answer, I marked the "D" response. Study the professor as well as the course material. Everything helps.

The moral of this story is not what you might think. Taking notes and listening to textbook tapes is the way to make good grades. This is true, but if you retain enough vision to outline a chapter in large print and read it, use that ability. Studying the professor also helps. Nonetheless, my point is this: I was learning how to learn by hearing, and I was retaining the knowledge. Thereafter, learning by hearing became even more effective. I used my eyes whenever I could as I worked on my degree. But the further I went, the more necessary it became to use my ears, and I came to trust them. Some students who are totally blind develop almost perfect recall. Residual vision distracts the partially sighted, but they can still develop listening and recall skills to a greater degree than persons with normal vision. The reason? They need those skills, whereas the person with normal vision does not.

Taking Tests

Reading and writing abilities determine how tests should be taken. Test taking calls for reading ability. The student must read the test, whether the questions are on a sheet of paper or on the black-board. The professor must then be able to read the student's answers. Not all of the test-taking methods discussed below will be appropriate for everyone, but everyone should find at least one that works for him or her. The list is not exhaustive. Do not be afraid to develop another way if needed.

Before each test, talk to the professor. Find out the format of the test and talk to him about your needs in taking it. Most professors are willing to accept whatever suggestion the student makes. Avoid any method that imposes on the professor or her time.

1. The professor can administer the test orally at a different time and place, with the student answering orally. For many people, this is the most stressful way to take a test, and many professors are reluctant to volunteer their time. Avoid this method if possible.

2. Take the test paper to a different room, where a reader reads the questions aloud, and then either the student or the reader writes the answers.

3. Take the test paper to a different room, where a reader reads the questions while the student dictates answers into a recorder. The professor then listens to the tape.

4. The student or reader reads the questions in a different room, and the student types the answers. Professors like this method. They prefer to read typed responses over hand-written ones, even if they are poorly typed.

5. The student or the reader reads the questions, and the student writes out answers on the blackboard in another room.

6. One of my professors suggested that on the day following the test I present a special report to the class. On that day, I taught the class (without notes) as my final exam.

7. The worst scenario is a printed test, where answers must be recorded in squares on a machine-readable answer sheet. In a situation like this, the reader must read the questions and mark the answer sheet. Another alternative is to go prepared with sheets of paper prenumbered in large print on the left

side of the page. Mark answers on the sheets in large print. Do not turn in these sheets. After completing the test, with the help of a friend or reader, transcribe answers to the proper machine-readable answer sheet.

8. If the test is timed, students who are visually impaired should not be forced to compete with students who have normal vision. Of course, most tests have built-in time limits — the class period ends and the room must be vacated for the next class. Discuss time limits for test taking with the professor. Generally, he will allow more time than he does for other students.

Most colleges and graduate schools require entrance exams. In almost all cases, these tests have time limits, and the visually impaired are in competition with all other students. As a rule, the visually impaired don't stand a chance under these circumstances unless concessions are made.

When standardized tests were developed, they were "normalized" by having thousands of students take them. In this way, average, above average, and below average test scores were determined. Student scores are compared to these norms. Most of these tests have "untimed norms" as well. Disabled students take the test without time limits, and officials score it against the untimed norms. Statisticians have balanced the timed and untimed norms. Scores on one are totally compatible with the other. The people administering the test will know about these untimed norms and about the provision for students to take the test without time limits. Before taking one of these exams, let the test officials know days in advance that special testing procedures need to be arranged.

Never walk into a test without knowing well in advance what the test format will be and how to cope with it.

Keyboard and Computer Skills

Typing is a skill the visually impaired should have. It isn't a requirement, but it makes life a lot easier. The pen is still our basic survival tool; language and reading are still king. But today, print is being displayed in a different way. In Chapter 24, I described large-print computers and software that enlarges computer screens. The visually impaired will find college work easier if they master keyboard skills and the use of computers.

Laser printers can transform anything prepared with any word-processing software into large print. With a computer equipped with large-print display capability, dictated class notes become large-print notes.

CHAPTER 34

Driving with Telescopic Glasses: An Introduction[4]

The average person with low vision who is fitted with telescopic glasses for driving receives little, if any, training in their use. As a result, users struggle to learn on their own. The end product is often a driver who lacks confidence and imposes limitations on where or when he drives.

The situation would be different if the patient were taught how to use the glasses. He must also become aware of the particular variables related to driving with telescopic glasses. If he follows a well-constructed training program with the help of a friend, the result should be a driver who finds no need for self-imposed restrictions.

This chapter presents the basic information needed by the driver who is partially sighted. The next chapter presents a training program closely tied to the variables involved in driving with telescopic glasses.

Basic Techniques

The partially sighted do not use their telescopic glasses constantly while driving. They drive primarily using their residual vision. The telescope(s) is merely an aid used occasionally to assist a person with diminished vision. The scope is used about 10 percent of the time. The other 90 percent of the time, the visually impaired drive without the scope.

The importance of this point cannot be overstressed, so despite the risk of redundancy, I will state it another way. With exceptions that will become obvious later, for the most part, the driver who is partially sighted uses residual vision to watch road conditions in the current block. The telescope scans conditions in the block beyond.

Telescopic glasses (sometimes called bioptic glasses) perform two different functions. First, they scan distant terrain. Second, they spot specific targets. Let's consider these functions separately.

Scanning

Scanning is using the telescope to survey traffic conditions one hundred yards or more ahead. The bioptic user moves the head in the shape of a square-bottomed "U." The chin moves down to align the scope on terrain at the left of the roadway. In a residential area, this would be the front yards of homes on the left. The head rotates to the right, sweeping the street ahead until the front yards on the right side of the road come into view. The chin then lifts, moving the scope out of the way, and the driver returns to using residual vision. (Some people prefer to make this sweeping move-ment from right to left.)

The purpose of the scanning movement is to spot situations or hazards in the block ahead. The bioptic user sees hundreds of things during each scanning movement. Children are playing in a yard near the street. A stop sign or traffic signal is visible at a distant intersection. A driver up ahead is executing a dangerous maneuver. The list is almost endless. The driver identifies all objects seen. They are either hazardous or routine. The bioptic user files these data in memory until the next scanning movement. Any differences or changes in the situation seen during the next scanning movement forewarn that some action may be required. **The primary function of scanning is to identify every object on or near the roadway ahead.**

Spotting

During scanning movements, one sees objects that cannot be identified. For example, while driving down a country road, a dark object is seen beside the road. It might be a mailbox on a wide stand. It could be a child. It could also be the south end of a northbound cow. The scope user sees the object, but cannot identify it. This is where spotting comes into play.

Spotting identifies "unknowns" picked up during scanning movements. To "spot" an object, the user sharply drops the chin straight down to align the scope on that one specific object. Once the unknown is identified, the chin lifts straight up to move the telescope out of the way. All drivers with partial vision must master this spotting technique. Learning to "hit" a given target immediately, without searching for it, takes practice, but mastering this skill is necessary if one is to drive safely.

Under normal driving conditions, spotting movements are executed leisurely. On occasion, however, one must spot targets very quickly. One should strive to develop sufficient skill to perform the entire spotting movement in one-half second or less.

Difficult Versus Easy Streets

Most new drivers quickly learn that it is more difficult to drive on some streets than on others. This holds true for the partially sighted as well. Many new drivers attribute the difficulty to the amount of traffic on a street. While this assessment may be true, it is not the only variable involved.

If certain factors are constant — such as the power of the scope(s) being used, the driver's visual acuity, the available light, and the light source and its relative position to the driver — then the difficulty of driving a given street involves three other variables: the number of things to be identified, visual clutter, and speed. The driver with low vision must understand these variables and how to control them if he or she is to drive safely without self-imposed restrictions. Let's look at each separately.

The Number of Things to Be Identified

On any given street, there are a specific number of things that must be seen and identified before the street can be driven safely. The things that must be seen include: other vehicles both parked and moving, cyclists, traffic signals, stop signs and a variety of other signs, pedestrians, and children playing near the road.

One must see or identify these things if one is to drive safely. **Identify** is stressed. The driver with partial vision sees a car. He can't tell whether it is a Ford or a Chevrolet, but he identifies the object as a car. He sees a cyclist; he can't tell whether it's a male or a female, but does it matter? He identifies the object as a cyclist. In like manner, a baseball rolls into the street. This driver might improperly call it a tennis ball, but what matters is that he sees a ball and it signals danger. A child could follow it into the street.

To drive safely, one must have object vision. If the patient with low vision still enjoys object vision, she is able to drive safely without normal definitive vision. One exception readily comes to mind. States adopt certain visual acuity levels for licensing drivers.

Having established the standard, they post highway and street signs of a size requiring that visual acuity to read them at a specific distance. This highlights one of the uses for the scope.

When first seen during scanning movements, every sign is an unknown, because it is too far away to be read. A few seconds later, the user spots and reads it, since she will have a visual acuity through the scope equivalent to that of routinely licensed drivers.

Almost all objects are identified ahead during scanning movements. Things not identified initially are identified a moment later, using the spotting technique. The number of objects to be identified is one factor in determining how difficult it will be to drive a given street.

Visual Clutter

The second variable involved is visual clutter. Visual clutter does not have to be seen to drive safely, but it interferes with the task of identifying objects that **must** be seen.

Consider a man standing beside interstate highway 10 where it crosses the desert in Arizona. In this environment, he stands out and is easily seen and identified. Place this man on a residential street with a ten-foot-tall bush behind him, and he becomes much more difficult to see. The bush is visual clutter. Other objects that can be classified as visual clutter are trees, utility poles with wires hanging down over the street, store signs, and similar objects near the street. These items do not need to be seen to drive safely, but they interfere with the process of identifying important things.

Speed

I have talked with many drivers who have partial vision, both those who use telescopic glasses and those who drive illegally without them. These people are keenly aware of their vision loss and of the public's fear of a "blind driver." They share a common denominator. **They all drive with their brains in gear.** They do not drive casually. They are alert to what is going on around them. They are certain that if something goes wrong and they have an accident, they will be blamed whether it was their fault or not. This hyper-awareness works to the benefit of the driver with partial vision.

While driving along in a comfortable situation, a person may gradually become aware that he is having to "rush" to keep up with conditions ahead. In other words, the number of things he needs to see and identify in order to drive safely has grown too large, given the amount of visual clutter in the area.

Reducing one's speed provides more time to identify all the objects ahead. This is exactly how to control both visual clutter and the number of objects one must identify. When the bioptic user feels he is getting behind or having to rush, he simply reduces speed. An automobile traveling sixty miles per hour covers eighty-eight feet per second. Cutting the speed to thirty doubles the time required to identify objects. However, it isn't necessary to slow to a speed hazardous to other traffic. Merely reducing speed five or ten miles per hour provides enough time to "catch up."

State-Imposed Restrictions

Once these three variables are understood, the restrictions commonly placed on bioptic users by licensing agencies make little sense. State authorities commonly restrict the licenses of bioptic users to stipulate no more than forty-five miles per hour, no highway driving, and no night driving. A restriction prohibiting driving on city freeways is justifiable, **but only for beginners learning to use their scopes.**

Consider highway driving. Compared to city driving, highway driving presents fewer things to see and identify. There is also far less visual clutter. Two-lane highways pose more difficulty than multiple-lane controlled-access roadways, but neither is as difficult as driving a thirty-five-mile-per-hour city street!

Advocates who support the use of the bioptic for driving debate whether these drivers should drive at night. I will make one comment concerning this argument. Driving familiar streets at night is only slightly more difficult than driving during daylight hours. About the only difference is that the driver will use the scope either more or less often at night than she does during the day. Whether she uses it more or uses it less depends on the condition that destroyed her vision. For example, some albinos see better at night and therefore will use the scope less.

Low-vision specialists disagree concerning the subject of driving at night with the bioptic. Some reject the idea completely. Since my vision has changed over the years, I have experience driving with various visual acuities. Possibly my experience can provide information on this controversy.

When my visual acuity was 20/60 to 20/120, I drove at night with little effort. I drove in strange cities, on city freeways, and on highways. Night driving required a slightly higher level of concentration, but it was not difficult. I began driving with a 2.2X Galilean scope and later changed to a 4X Galilean. With the 4X Galilean, driving at night immediately became difficult, because the $4^1/_2$-degree field with the 4X was too narrow. When I changed to using a 6X prismatic scope with a $7^1/_2$-degree field, the ease of night driving returned.

Today, with a visual acuity of 20/240, and using the 6X prismatic scope, I can still drive highways, strange cities, and freeways, but I am not completely comfortable driving at night.

A driver's comfort and discomfort are good indicators of where or if he should be allowed to drive.

Familiar Versus Unfamiliar Streets

The three variables — number of things to identify, visual clutter, and speed — also explain why it is easier to drive familiar streets than unfamiliar ones. Obviously, on a well-known street there are fewer things to identify. Read a specific sign a number of times. How many times does it take to memorize it? On familiar streets, drivers know the speed limit and where it changes. They know the location of traffic signals and stop signs, so no time is "lost" looking for them. The elimination of these tasks from the busy bioptic user's schedule makes driving familiar streets no more complicated than it is for drivers with normal vision.

Speedometers and Traffic Signals

Once a driver learns the basic techniques of using the scope(s), he or she will develop his or her own individualized driving habits and techniques, but advice in two areas may prove helpful.

Speedometers

The average user of the bioptic cannot read a speedometer. The indicator or needle is visible, but the numbers are not. There are at least three ways to deal with this.

1. Memorize the speedometer using a magnifier. When the needle is at nine o'clock, your speed might be thirty miles per hour. At twelve o'clock, it might be forty-five. If you cannot see the needle, take the car to a speedometer-repair

shop and ask them to install a wider needle in a visible color.
When the needle is visible, you can judge speed by needle
position.

2. Paint the speedometer face, dividing it into color-coded
    wedges. I have taken speedometers out and painted the
    wedge between thirty and forty-five either yellow or white. I
    painted the wedge between fifty-five and sixty-five the same
    way. The painted segments on the face greatly assist in esti-
    mating speed by needle position.

3. When driving on the highway, I use two techniques. When
    the needle is positioned approximately at the desired speed, I
    set the cruise control. I momentarily slip a "reading cap" onto
    the scope. This changes the scope's focal length to about
    eighteen inches, so I can read the speedometer clearly. I then
    adjust my speed as necessary and reset the cruise control.
    With the speed set, I can forget about the speedometer.

Some newer automobiles feature large-print digital speedometers.
Some bioptic users can read these without special aids. Simply bend
down briefly to get closer.

Traffic Lights

Immediately after passing through an intersection on an unfamiliar
street, scan the next intersection, looking for the location of traffic
signals or stop signs. On familiar streets, omit this step. When you're
about one-half block from the light, quickly spot it to determine its
color. If it is red or amber, prepare to stop. If it is green, continue,
but anticipate a change to amber. Depending on your speed, there is
a point where you have time to stop should the light change. At this
"go or no go" point, quickly spot the light again. If the light is still

green, lift your chin to move the scope out of the way and drive through the intersection, using only your eyeballs. Never use the scope beyond this "go or no go" point. Never drive through an intersection using the scope. This is "eyeball country," and one is near enough to the things that must be seen that the scope isn't needed anyway.

Learning to Drive

The next chapter gives a detailed training program for driving with telescopic glasses. The program assumes that the trainees are experienced drivers who, for some reason, have lost some of their vision. People who are not experienced drivers and are learning to drive and use their bioptic at the same time have a more difficult task, though not as difficult as you might think.

If this is your situation, I recommend learning to operate a vehicle without wearing telescopic glasses. Drive with a friend. Let her report on things that would be seen in the scope. She can read the signs and watch distant road conditions. Such a routine will quickly teach you why the scope is needed, and for what.

Most cities of fifty thousand people or more have a part of the city devoted to warehouses, light manufacturing, and the like. These areas are virtually deserted on Sundays — a good place and time to gain street-driving experience. Those living in cities smaller than this will find lightly traveled residential areas where driving is also easier.

Two Scopes or One?

I have used both single scopes and binocular configurations for driving. In highway driving, twin scopes are fine, even in the constant use configuration, where a driver uses the scopes all the time. When it comes to city driving, a single scope in spotting configuration is much more versatile. For example, while sitting at a traffic light waiting for it to change, the scope points at the light. There is a ring-shaped blind spot or scotoma around the field of view through the scope (I will say more about this later). With twin scopes, the scotoma blots out the entire intersection, reaching down to the hood of the car. The traffic light is all one can see. The scotoma obliterates the rest of the intersection.

When the light changes, the driver raises his chin, lifting the scopes out of the way to see the intersection. If it is clear, he continues. In the meantime, the guy behind is blowing his horn. When a single scope is used, the scope sees the light, but the off eye sees the intersection continuously, so there is no delay in driving through the intersection.

There is a learning process in using one scope. Both eyes are kept open, but the image from the off eye is suppressed. Generally, the visually impaired have one eye that is better than the other. This makes suppressing the off eye easy to learn.

About the Scope and Glasses

In this book I have urged you to combine coping techniques whenever possible. For example, I suggest using both light and contrast enhancement, along with getting closer. It is wise to do the same with driving glasses. I recommend the following.

The carrier lenses made by Designs for Vision are plastic. Have these carrier lenses dyed amber, for contrast enhancement. Not all low-vision specialists do this, but there are optical companies in most fairly large cities that provide the service.

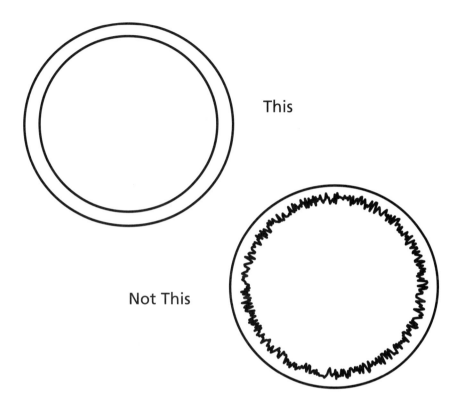

This

Not This

Figure 34.1: Checking the Scope

When looking through the scope, it appears that the scope's "housing" is visible around the field seen through the scope. When the glasses fit correctly, the inside edge of this housing appears sharp and clear. If the inner edge is blurred, move the glasses closer to the eye.

If you won't be using the glasses to drive at night, have the lenses dyed to match the lightest shade of amber provided by Corning. Most optical companies will know what shade this is. If they don't, they can find out by calling Corning. (Find the phone number in Appendix B.) If the glasses will be used at night, the lenses should be lighter than this. Dyeing them about half as dark as Corning's light amber should be fine. Of course, if the user suffers from albinism or is otherwise very light sensitive, it may be necessary to use a darker shade of amber. Run tests to determine the shade needed. Don't have the glasses tinted just any color.

The scope, which contains several lenses, does not need to be tinted. Each clear lens filters out 10 percent of the light. Rarely will people find they have problems with the scope, even if they are very light sensitive.

Some low-vision specialists fit NOIR amber sunglasses over telescopic glasses. They cut a hole in the sunglasses for the scope. This procedure works, but tinted lenses are a less cumbersome aid.

The proper fitting of telescopic glasses is important. If the scope is too far from the eye, it restricts the field of view. There is a simple way to determine that the glasses fit correctly, but the doctor must depend on user feedback to do this. If the scope is the proper distance from the eye, the full view through the scope will be clear and sharp. If the glasses are too far from the eyes, the outer area of the field will appear fuzzy. If your vision is not clear all the way to the outside, pull the glasses closer to your eyes to see if it clears up. If it does, ask the doctor to move the glasses closer. My eyelashes are fairly long, and I have threatened at times to cut them off my left eye. My scope needs to be very close, and sometimes my lashes touch it. See Figure 34.1 for more details.

I strongly recommend that telescopic glasses not be fitted in the doctor's office. Go to the lobby where they can be tested using better light and distant targets.

CHAPTER 35

Driving with Telescopic Glasses: A Training Program[5]

This training program grows out of variables that affect one's driving, as discussed in the previous chapter. A trainee should only undertake the training program after reading and understanding the foundation upon which it rests.

Rationale and Structure of the Training Program

I frequently criticize traffic engineers for the placement of traffic signals and "one way" street signs. Nevertheless, the same engineers prove amazingly consistent in assigning speed limits to city streets that reflect the two variables — **number of things to be identified** and **visual clutter.** As the posted speed limit increases, there are fewer things to identify and there is less visual clutter.

Since this is true, it might seem logical to begin driver training on a roadway with a posted speed limit of seventy miles per hour and continue progressively to a street posted twenty-five miles per hour. The training program that follows does not follow such a progression because of the third variable — **speed.**

In addition, the relative importance of the three variables changes according to the conditions found on each type of roadway. The amount of weight to assign each variable, to produce a training program that goes from the simple to the more difficult, is strictly a matter of judgment. Having driven over seven hundred thousand miles using bioptic glasses, I assume that my experience qualifies me to make these judgments.

The Training Program

In driving with telescopic glasses, personality variables are as important as vision itself. The most important variable is self-confidence. We gain self-confidence through success. We lose confidence through failure. In executing the training program outlined in this chapter, it is vitally important to follow the steps one at a time. Stay with each step until you feel completely comfortable and proficient at that level. Especially when the phase titled "In-Car Training" begins, the trainee should practice each step until fully comfortable. Then repeat each step on other streets posted with the same speed limit.

Many people have requested copies of this training program. Some ask me to rush a copy to them since they plan to take their driving test in a week or so. Let me make clear that no one can complete this program in a week or so. Learning occurs outside the car, not in it. The in-car experience constitutes data collection. Learning takes place later, when drivers assimilate the data and add it to what they already know.

Because of individual differences, it is impossible to judge how long a person will require to complete the program, but one step per week is a fair estimate, assuming the driver is practicing twice per week.

A. Target Practice

Step 1. From a stationary base, learn to spot stationary targets.

Procedure: Stand on the front porch or in the yard and use the spotting technique to spot targets no closer than one-half block away. Try for accuracy at first, not speed. Face the target; drop the chin straight down to "hit" the target with the scope. Identify the target, then lift the chin straight up. If you miss the target, lift the chin and try again. **Do not turn the head right or left, looking for the missed target.** You must learn to hit the target accurately and almost immediately without searching for it.

Once you achieve accuracy, try spotting targets directly across the street. Closer targets require greater accuracy. When you hit targets consistently on the first try, work on speed. The objective is to learn to do this in one-half second and from a moving car.

You do not need this degree of skill before beginning in-car training, but understand that experienced bioptic users make these spotting movements in well under one-half second. Continue to work on both speed and accuracy.

Step 2. From a stationary base, spot and track moving targets.

Procedure: Stand about a block from and perpendicular to a busy street. Spot and track specific vehicles. Pick out a specific vehicle using the eyeballs, then quickly spot it with the scope, then turn the head, keeping it in view in the scope.

When you consistently achieve success, move closer to the street. Notice that the nearer the target, the faster the head must turn to track the target. The ability to spot and track low-flying birds and high-flying aircraft defines a skill greater than what is needed for driving, but having this skill level is worth the effort!

B. In-Car Training (Before Driving)

Step 3. From a moving base, spot stationary targets.

Step 4. From a moving base, spot and track moving targets.

Procedure: Those who live in a city with a "loop" highway around it have an excellent roadway for this training. If there is no loop, use a highway in a rural or suburban area.

Ride as a passenger in a car driven by a friend. First, learn to spot stationary targets like barns, specific trees, or houses about one-half mile off the road. Hit these targets on the first try. Turning the head to locate a missed target is not good enough. Notice that targets one-half mile away require "tracking," because the car is moving. The closer the target, the faster the head must turn.

Next, concentrate on targets closer to the highway, including signs to read. Once targets are hit more often than missed, try spotting vehicles moving perpendicular to the highway. Find opportunity for this training at overpasses, where the highway crosses above another street.

During both steps 3 and 4, occasionally try a scanning movement, looking at traffic conditions no less than one-half mile ahead. Note: when driving on a controlled-access highway — one where there is no cross traffic and no traffic lights — scanning movements need not involve much left to right movement of the head. The field of view through the scope(s) is wide enough that spotting-like movements can be substituted and used to examine conditions one-half mile to one mile ahead. **This exception is not true for farm-to-market roads and two-lane highways.** Wider scanning movements are needed to see traffic crossing highways that are not controlled access.

C. In-Car Training (Driving)

Step 5. Drive on a controlled-access highway.

Procedure: As with any other training program, begin with the simplest task and then go to the more difficult. This means that your first in-car experience should be driving on a controlled-access highway (a highway having no cross traffic or traffic lights). This is the easiest of all driving environments.

Choose a clear, dry Sunday morning. Avoid holiday-season traffic. Have your friend drive twenty miles out of town to a controlled-access highway.

The highway must be a four-lane roadway as a minimum requirement. Know in advance where to exit. The exit should be well away from town. Don't select a highway that passes through a town unless the town is very small. Avoid any highway with toll-booths. These parameters define a roadway carrying minimal traffic. On such a roadway, the number of things to identify is minimal. Visual clutter is minimal.

For the most part, you have only two visual tasks to perform: (1) stay in the outside lane (use eyeballs for this, not the scope), and (2) don't run into the car ahead.

Select a safe location to change places with your friend. Get behind the wheel, and with his help, drive onto the highway. Accelerate to forty-five miles per hour. Every ten seconds or so, make a scanning movement with the scope to view traffic conditions one-half mile to one mile ahead.

Do not pass a sign without identifying it. Don't read the sign; identify it. A sign saying "Throwing…" need not be read in its entirety. It concerns littering, which has nothing to do with safe driving. Identify, don't read, every sign.

There are hundreds of signs providing information or warnings that have little bearing on safe driving. With experience, you will be able to give these signs a cursory glance and then ignore them. If you do not "waste time" reading unnecessary signs, you have more time to concentrate on the road and on important signs. Signs are made in different shapes and colors. Save time by learning what these shapes and colors mean.

Don't rush it, but once you feel comfortable, increase speed. Go to fifty, then sixty. Stay at each speed until fully comfortable with it. Finally, increase speed up to seventy mph.

When you reach a place close to your selected exit (you will see the exit while scanning), reduce speed and spot the exit from about a hundred yards. A white line on the right marks the right margin of the highway. At the exit, this line curves to the right, following the exit ramp. Beyond the exit, the white line appears again, joined by the line marking the left side of the exit ramp. These two lines converge and form a point. See Figure 35.1.

This point is a steering marker. When exiting right, steer to the right of the point. When continuing down the highway, steer to the left of the point. All bioptic users should "spot" each of the exit "points" they pass when driving on the highway. Exits are often confusing, and use of these points will ensure that things are well under control.

After you exit, cross to the other side of the highway, and drive back the opposite way. Stop and switch places with your friend long before you reach even moderate traffic conditions.

On the trip out, your friend should sit sideways in the seat and give warning when traffic comes from behind. On the return trip, start using the car's mirrors to track traffic to the rear. Looking ahead, a visually impaired driver can see well enough to drive safely for a certain distance without the scope. Beyond that point,

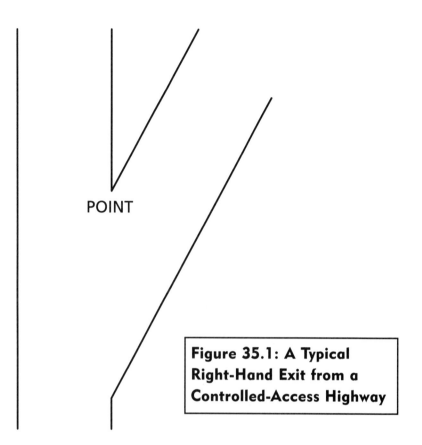

POINT

Figure 35.1: A Typical Right-Hand Exit from a Controlled-Access Highway

she uses the scope for greater definitive power. The rearview mirrors work the same way. In the mirror, drivers can see the same distance behind as they can see forward. When targets are "out of range" for eyeballs in the mirror, spot the mirror with the scope.

Repeat this exercise until you feel no stress. One to two hours in one session should be sufficient to proceed to the next step.

Step 6. Drive on a 25–30 mph residential street.

Procedure: The next training ground is a residential area composed of single-family homes, where the speed limit is twenty-five to thirty miles per hour.

Residential areas contain excessive visual clutter, such as bushes and trees, but slow driving speeds allow time to see and identify everything. In a residential area, the partially sighted driver will be unable to see as far ahead as he did on the highway. Visual clutter limits how far down the road the driver can see.

Make scanning movements, sweeping well into front yards on both sides of the street. Know what hazards relate to each type of street. Look for these hazards. In a residential area, expect to see pedestrians, pets, cyclists, and children playing. On a rural road, expect to find a cow wandering down the shoulder. Anticipating what you **might** see will help you identify objects first seen as unknowns.

Curved streets are more difficult than straight ones. A curved street limits your view down the road. Until this training program is completed, avoid selecting training ground that includes curved streets.

Again, when comfortable and confident, go on to the next step.

Step 7. Drive on a 45–55 mph major traffic artery.

Procedure: From the residential area, the trainee moves to the major thoroughfare — the next level of difficulty. The speed is much faster, but there is far less visual clutter than was found in residential areas. **Note: a forty-five to fifty-five mph street does not mean a city freeway.**

Maintain appropriate speed. Drive no less than ten miles per hour below the posted limit. As in step 5, be selective about the day of the week and time of day. Avoid rush-hour traffic.

Practice at this level until your speed in using the scope gives you enough confidence to keep pace with other traffic. Turn off this street well before the speed limit reduces to forty mph.

Step 8. Drive on a 40 mph residential street.

Procedure: On this street the speed is lower than in step 7, but there is more visual clutter. Carefully select the street as well as the day of the week and time of day.

Select a place to enter this street from a residential street. Leave this street well before reaching an area with a speed limit of thirty-five mph. As before, become perfectly comfortable driving this type of street before moving to step 9.

Step 9. Drive during downtown rush-hour traffic.

Procedure: This training area involves less difficulty than areas already mastered. People commonly think driving difficulty increases with the number of cars in the area. This is a psychological barrier a driver must overcome. Driving isn't more difficult at slow speeds, only more frustrating. **Other cars actually aid the driving process.** Bioptic users need to discover how and why this is true.

Select a weekday, and have your friend drive downtown. Choose a location to trade places with the friend where merging with traffic isn't too difficult. In most cities, 4:30 P.M. will be about right.

The precise conditions desired are bumper-to-bumper traffic, traveling thirty miles per hour or slower. As orientation, let your friend drive around a planned route. The training ground should be a rectangular area about four blocks long and one block wide. Drive around this rectangle during rush hour, making right turns.

Spend an hour going around this rectangle, staying in the right lane all the time. There are many things to see and identify, but the trainee will rarely need the scope. Other cars make it obvious when a traffic light has changed, but practice spotting the lights anyway.

If you are first in line at a light, point the scope at the light. Wait for the light to change, check for pedestrians, and then continue. Driving here is easy. Remember the basic rules: Stay in the outside lane and don't hit the car ahead. Could anything be simpler?

Be alert to the characteristics of the area where you are driving. Pedestrians may be coming into the street to enter parked cars. Keep an eye on them. If they or their car doors extend into the outside lane, stop. Do not change lanes and go around them.

This exercise assumes good spotting skills. The only targets for the scope are traffic signals. All other things are close enough to be seen with the eyeballs. This makes driving here very easy. **A tip: When using the scope(s) to spot signals in traffic, make sure to include part of the car ahead in the scope's field of view. If possible, pick up a taillight. This gives instant warning if the car ahead stops.**

Other cars will be bumper to bumper. As a beginning bioptic user, wisely maintain more distance between cars than other drivers do. Follow the rule used in driver-education courses: never get so close to the car ahead that you cannot see its rear tires.

Step 10. Drive on a 35 mph street.

Procedure: Streets with a speed limit of thirty-five miles per hour present one of the most difficult driving tasks one can experience. (The other is city freeways during rush-hour traffic.) Characteristically, these are commercial areas with storefronts fairly close to the street. There may be parallel or diagonal parking at the curb and substantial vehicular traffic. Store signs jutting out to the curb are common.

There are many things to identify; on top of that, this is an area with excessive visual clutter. Pick a day of the week and time of day to avoid heavy traffic.

In this area, anticipate pedestrians and cars pulling out into the street from the curb.

D. Expanding Potential

Step 11. Mix it up.

Procedure: Up to this point, the trainee has specialized. He started with a specific type of street and stayed with it. Each type of street had its unique hazards and targets that the driver anticipated seeing. In other words, there was a mental set associated with each. The driver anticipated finding a given type of hazard on each one. By contrast, driving around in random areas calls for the trainee to shift mental gears when going from one type of street to the next. However, describing the process is far more difficult than doing it.

Go out and have a ball. Drive around town going from one type of street to the other. While enjoying your new freedom, remember that the partially sighted **never drive casually.** Keep your attention levels up and conversation down.

Step 12. Drive on a four-lane highway (not controlled access).

Procedure: This is easy driving, because passing other cars is no problem. Scanning becomes very important, because you're looking a long way ahead for cross traffic entering the highway and traffic lights. There is less visual clutter than in most areas already mastered. Speed is no problem. There probably isn't a minimal speed posted.

Stay in the right lane at forty-five miles per hour until comfortable, then accelerate to fifty-five. Anticipate cross traffic and traffic signals.

Note: the remaining two steps in the program need not be taken immediately. Some drivers will want to accumulate more driving experience before proceeding to the final two steps.

Step 13. Drive on a two-lane highway.

Procedure: These highways typically have narrow shoulders and follow the contour of the land. Driving here is not difficult. As a beginner, follow the rules already mentioned several times. Stay in the right lane and don't hit the car ahead. The challenge here is passing other cars. At first, let your friend help you judge distance. Learn that passing can be done safely.

When passing, maintain your position on the road **using your eyeballs.** Use the scope to assure that it is clear to pass. Once in the passing lane, use spotting movements every other second to see if traffic is coming. Here, spotting skill pays off. Use the following three-second method when passing.

The **first second,** use your eyeballs to look at lane lines to avoid veering out of the lane.

The **next second,** use the scope to spot the horizon.

The **third second,** return to the use of your eyeballs, viewing lane lines.

Continue changing from eyeballs to scope until passing is accomplished. On level terrain this isn't too difficult. A driver can see far enough ahead to know the highway is clear. The major problem is simply staying in the lane.

In hilly country, passing becomes more difficult. The next hill limits vision and passing time. This situation may call for ten or more changes from eyeballs to scope during a five-second interval.

Gradually, a trainee learns to judge distance through the scope(s). This isn't the kind of judgment that says, "That car is 150 yards down the road." Rather, it is the assurance that there is room and time enough to pass safely.

Step 14. Drive on a city freeway.

Procedure: The difficulty level of driving city freeways is not great. There is very little visual clutter, and while there are many things to see and identify, most of them are other automobiles headed in the same direction. The problem here is psychological. Other drivers will whip from lane to lane, jockeying for position. They will tailgate. They will suddenly cut across lanes to make an exit they are about to miss. Seeing these things increases your awareness of danger and creates a feeling of discomfort. Overcome these feelings by developing confidence in your own skill. With experience it becomes easier.

After a time, the bioptic user will confidently change lanes and pull around slow-moving trucks without easing up on the accelerator. **A bioptic user must never tailgate.** When someone cuts into the space ahead of you, ease off the accelerator and restore the interval desired.

Your first experience driving on a freeway might be a Sunday around 10:00 A.M. or 2:00 P.M. To begin with, stay in the outside lane and know in advance where to exit. For your second practice session, choose a weekday at the same time. By the third session, you will begin to realize that this driving isn't difficult.

Freeway driving is mostly eyeball country. The scope has limited use here. Use it to scan for trouble well ahead and for locating exits. The situation is like driving downtown during rush-hour traffic. The difference is speed.

E. Graduation

Graduation for the bioptic user involves more than driving solo. State law probably controls when you will drive solo. This isn't as important as having confidence in your newly acquired skills. In the fullest sense, graduation from this school means independent mobility — the ability to drive without reservation.

Several times during the above training program, I stated, "Stay in the right lane" or "Hold down your speed." Graduation means not having to rely on these crutches. It means driving anywhere a person with normal vision can drive and at the same speed. As a trainee, you are still a learner and will continue to learn for many years. But the skills you have learned thus far should equip you to drive where and when you wish.

Since confidence in one's driving skills is one of the most important variables related to driving with the bioptic, keep your confidence high by driving often. Driving only occasionally erodes confidence.

CHAPTER 36

Misconceptions about Driving with Telescopic Glasses

Earlier I referred to the battle being waged concerning use of the bioptic. This "war" has gone on for years and isn't yet resolved.

Frequently, professional journals in the field of visual impairment publish articles related to driving with the bioptic. Often, writers who oppose their use focus on some new reason why the bioptic is unsafe.

Opponents of the bioptic for driving often use the phrase "inherent optical deficiencies" to describe it's limitations. Some of their observations are correct. Telescopes do have built-in restrictions. The real question is, do these "inherent deficiencies" have anything to do with driving safety?

Generally, objections to the use of the bioptic come from people who, I believe, are detached from the reality, and who offer theoretical objections. I often match the reality of my seven hundred thousand miles of driving with the bioptic against these prognostications.

Each time I have challenged opponents, my experience has poked holes in their theories, and some have admitted this. Others try to explain away my experience by saying, "He has been lucky." Many imply that I am an exception, unlike other drivers with visual impairment who couldn't possibly match my performance. I wish it were true! I could get used to the title of Superman. Alas, it isn't true. Thousands of people, of all ages, drive safely with the bioptic. If I am a Superman, then we must all be called Supermen and Wonder Women.

Those who drive with the bioptic need to know about these so-called "inherent deficiencies," because some carry an element of truth. If the scope is used improperly, the criticisms against it sometimes prove valid.

A good example of an article condemning the use of the bioptic is "Bioptic Telescopic Spectacles and Driving Performance: A Study in Texas," by O. Lippmann, A. L. Corn, and M. C. Lewis, published in The Journal of Visual Impairment and Blindness, May 1988. Dr. Otto Lippmann is a retired ophthalmologist who served as chairman of the Medical Advisory Board in Texas for many years. Anne Corn, Doctor of Special Education, worked for the University of Texas in Austin when I first met her. M. C. Lewis is unknown to me.

About Statistical Analysis

Using statistical techniques, the writers above "matched" a group of persons having normal vision with a group of people having visual impairment who drive with telescopic glasses. The results showed that the partially sighted group had a significantly higher accident rate than the "normalized" group.

While earning my doctor's degree, I took four courses in statistics and two on experimental design. Professors frequently cautioned students about an error researchers commonly make. Finding that there is a statistical difference between two groups of humans does not prove there is a causal relationship to account for these differences.

Someone illustrated this point by doing a study that "proved" that the sale of liquor correlated significantly with the number of Southern Baptist ministers ordained during a given period. Readers probably know that most Southern Baptist ministers are teetotalers. Statistics can prove that the consumption of alcohol increased during the same period that ordinations increased, but that is all statistics can prove. Proving a statistical relationship between test groups isn't difficult; proving a **causal** relationship to account for differences or similarities is much more difficult. The consumption of alcohol and the ordination of ministers can increase at the same time, but this does not prove that ministers were responsible for the increased consumption.

A local Texas licensing-bureau chief once reported that 12 percent of drivers in Texas cause most of the accidents. These people continue to drive with a valid license until they cause four accidents during any twelve-month period.

My challenge to opponents of the bioptic is this: why not compare the bioptic users to this group of accident-prone persons who can drive hassle-free forever in Texas, causing three accidents per year for the rest of their lives. Is the driving of bioptic users as bad as this? Is it better, equal, or worse?

Time after time, research has proven that handicapped drivers drive more safely than drivers with no impairment. This is true for all types of disability, including visual. If opponents of the bioptic are truly interested in public safety, maybe they should stop wasting time keeping the bioptic driver off the road. They should spend more time controlling those who can pass the vision test but who lack other, more important qualifications for driving.

Finding that bioptic users have more accidents than a normalized control group doesn't prove a causal relationship between these accidents and the "inherent optical deficiencies" of the scope.

Listed below are some of the major "inherent optical deficiencies" that opponents of the bioptic talk about. Put them to the test of reality.

The Ring Scotoma

At one time, I made a list of seventeen different objections I had heard expressed to driving with the bioptic. Among them was the fact that they cause a sore neck. It is true. Muscles seldom used are employed using the bioptic. When the bioptic is first used, these muscles will complain. This is strictly a temporary problem and has nothing to do with driving safety.

Consider the figures presented by the Lippmann article mentioned above. The 3X Galilean scope provides a 6-degree field of view, and the 3X prismatic provides a 12-degree field. Around this field of clear vision lies an area encompassing 12 to 15 degrees of total blindness caused by the scope housing and the nature of telescopes. Let's examine the importance of this doughnut-shaped scotoma in driving.

The ring scotoma poses a threat to driving only if it is assumed that the user drives looking through the scope constantly, or that his neck is as inflexible as concrete.

Opponents of the bioptic refuse to believe that the scope is used only intermittently. Even if it were used constantly, a 12- to 15-degree turn of the head would cover the field defect. Most bioptic users do not use the telescope constantly. They use it occasionally. When the scope is not in use, the ring scotoma presents no problem.

If a user turns his head to aim the scope at a sign beside the road, the ring scotoma can blot out a semitrailer truck one block ahead. The truck was there in his field of vision (with or without the scope) before he used the scope to read the sign. Does he forget it is there during the instant it takes to identify the sign?

This segment of the article also implies the misconception that the ring scotoma blots out all of one's peripheral vision. Each eye provides a visual field of about 150 degrees: 90 degrees to the outside of the point of fixation, and about 60 degrees to the inside. (The nose blocks off about 30 degrees to the inside.) Begin with the 6 degrees for the scope's field, and add to it a factor of two times the 12 to 15 degrees on either side of the scope's field. This gives a total of 36 degrees. That leaves 114 degrees of one's peripheral vision (in one eye) actively performing its function. In short, the ring scotoma does not blot out all peripheral vision, as implied.

If low-vision specialists fit only one telescope in glasses used for driving, as I believe they should, the whole matter of the ring scotoma becomes a moot issue. In such a case, one eye is always free of field defects, even when the other eye uses the scope.

A Field of Six Feet Viewing Targets Fifty Feet Away

In the aforementioned article, the researchers write that the 3X scope offers a field of view the width of one car (six feet) at a distance of fifty feet. I have never used the 3X scope in question, but let's assume they are right. The researchers' assumption is that the bioptic driver is viewing things fifty feet away with the scope. Moreover, they imply that the driver **needs** the scope to see targets fifty feet away. Why would he use it on targets that close if it weren't needed?

There are only three situations when I view things fifty feet away through the scope. (1) While waiting for a light to change, I might find myself looking at a traffic signal fifty feet away or closer. (2) I might read a sign from this distance. (3) If an attractive lady crosses the intersection while I wait for a light to change, I **might** be tempted to get a better look by using the scope. It is important to remember that the telescope is a **distance-viewing** tool.

Eye-care professionals consider targets twenty feet away to be distance-viewing tasks. This is true, but distance-viewing tasks while driving means viewing targets no less than one-half block ahead; usually they are even farther than that. The scope is not used on targets twenty or even fifty feet away, because it isn't needed on targets that close.

When my visual acuity was 10/60 (20/120), I could see everything I needed to see out to two-tenths of a mile (about 350 yards) ahead without the scope. I could see every car. I couldn't identify them by make, but I could see them. I could see cyclists. I could see a cow (maybe it was a bull) that had escaped its pasture. I could see a hitchhiker alongside the road. I saw the signs, but I couldn't read them until I got closer. I didn't need the telescope inside 350 yards to see all I needed to see to drive safely on a highway.

If a driver has object-identification vision on an open highway for 350 yards or more, then she doesn't need the scope within this range. (The one exception would be reading the signs mentioned above.) The field of view through my 6X prismatic scope is $7^1/2$ degrees. Applied to driving, this field of view is more than seven lanes of traffic wide when viewing targets only one hundred yards away. (Note: this scope is the first in the series of Designs for Vision prismatic scopes that are not focusable. The current 6X focusable has a $6^1/2$ degree field.)

Now that my vision has dropped to 10/120 (20/240), I can't see as far down the highway as I did before; yet I see far enough to experience no problems. When I leave the highway and come into town, where visual clutter makes it more difficult to see well, the distance seen down the road shrinks in direct proportion to the amount of visual clutter present. I've driven under all conditions, and I've never found a situation where I couldn't see all I needed to see to drive safely in town. And of course in such a congested area, I drive at city speeds (like everyone else) so there is no need to see as far down the road.

The scope is used to see what a person cannot see with their own eyes. It is never used on targets inside eyeball distances; therefore, the impact of the argument against driving with a scope that sees only six feet wide on targets fifty feet away is lost. This point illustrates my contention that ophthalmologists know little about subnormal vision. They really don't know what the visually impaired can see at any distance.

Reading Highway Signs

Opponents of the bioptic make an issue of reading highway signs. The article under discussion says that it takes three seconds to read a six-word highway sign, and a quarter of a second for the bioptic user to shift from eyeballs to scope. They conclude, "The individual drives blind through traffic for 286 feet," since a car traveling at sixty mph covers eighty-eight feet per second.

What they are saying is that reading a sign off to the side of the road allows the ring scotoma to blot out the highway ahead, so the driver proceeds down the highway "blind" for 286 feet. This, of course, ignores the fact that the scope was used a moment before to clear the highway for a mile ahead.

I will make two points regarding this issue. Do people actually read all highway signs? I don't, at least not all of them. Signs are **identified,** but all "six words" need not be read. When an orange sign is seen ahead, it means caution or construction. The color of the sign tells me what I need to know. When I see an orange sign, I look down the road with the scope to find out what lies ahead. It isn't necessary to read every word of each sign.

A momentary glance identifies each sign as either information not needed or something that demands attention. I do not spend three and a quarter seconds studying the message.

Exceptions exist, of course, but routinely, signs are given a very short quarter-second look. What about that sign warning "BRIDGE OUT"? Do they put up signs saying "BRIDGE OUT" without barricading the road ahead? No.

Is this system viable? Experience proves it is. Most of my driving experience has been on highways. I have never encountered a problem caused by driving "blind through traffic for 286 feet while reading signs."

My second point is that using the words "through traffic" is employing scare tactics. I do not take my eyes off the road for three seconds to read a sign when cars around me are doing seventy miles per hour. In close traffic, my attention is riveted on nearby cars, and frankly, I assume each driver is drunk, insane, or blind!

I have explained how I drive as a partially sighted driver. Now consider what I do **not** do. Routinely, people with normal vision take their eyes off the road for more than $3^1/2$ seconds while talking to a passenger. They scrutinize things off the road for 5 or 6 seconds at a time. By contrast, all persons with visual impairment know their vision is defective, so they concentrate every part of that visual ability on the road. When my wife and I take a driving vacation, my wife sees the scenery. I see the road.

Decay of Visual Acuity Caused by Car Vibration

Many persons with partial vision, and even their doctors, find it inconceivable that they can perform some visual tasks better than persons with normal vision. Nonetheless, this is true. Place a person with normal vision on a city bus traveling over bumpy streets. Give him a strong telescope and ask him to read storefront signs. He will give up in frustration. Vibration destroys visual acuity for the normally sighted.

The partially sighted commonly use 8X and 10X scopes for this purpose, and I met one woman who used a 20X scope this way. As humans, we must learn how to see. When light enters the eye, it focuses on the retina. Light-sensing cells fire, and a coded electronic signal goes to the brain. Once the brain has learned what each code means, a person "sees." We "see" when our brains can find a match on file in our visual memory center for the code currently sent by the eye. When vibration distorts that signal, a person's normal vision deteriorates rapidly. The brain of a person who is partially sighted has apparently learned to cope with weak, fuzzy signals. This is the way he or she sees all the time! Regardless of the reason, it is a fact that persons with partial vision use telescopic aids of high power without serious decay of visual acuity. Car vibration does not adversely affect the driver using the bioptic. Only the normally sighted will have difficulty with this phenomenon.

Speed-Smear

Long before I'd heard of speed-smear, I had observed its reality while riding with my parents as a child. In an automobile, lock the head and eyes as if in a vise; look straight ahead, and images in peripheral fields blur as speed increases.

Opponents to the use of the bioptic for driving have computed that this speed-smear merges with the ring scotoma around the field seen through the bioptic. This means the bioptic user is driving with tunnel vision, seeing only objects visible through the scope.

You have experienced this effect and countered it the same way as the bioptic user. You turn your head to track objects to the side.

This is a valid argument against driving with the bioptic — but **only if** the bioptic is used improperly. Opponents assume the user is pointing the telescope straight down the highway, using it constantly, while his eyes, neck, and brain are locked in position. In fact, a driver uses the bioptic only about 10 percent of the time.

Speed-smear is only another theoretical objection, far removed from reality, based on incorrect assumptions.

The "Jack-in-the-Box Effect"

The "Jack-in-the-box effect" is another objection to the use of the bioptic for driving that assumes that the head and eyes are immobile and that the scope is used constantly.

Two ophthalmologists originated the term. They mounted a movie camera on a tripod, extended it through the sunroof of their car, and drove through town with the camera running. (One of the doctors gave this description in a trial conducted in Pittsburgh several years ago.) They say the film is an example of what a bioptic user sees as he drives. The film is frightening enough to scare fleas off a dog! Cars moving across traffic pop into the camera's field of view suddenly, without warning — hence the term "jack-in-the-box effect."

Other bioptic users and I have told critics that this film in no way represents reality, but the "experts" continue to use it. It reminds me of an old Texas saying I heard shortly after moving here in 1966: "When you run out of real ammunition, shoot blanks. At least they make noise!"

I have already discussed how scanning movements with the scope are used to survey the road ahead. Scanning movements, using either the scope or one's own eyeballs, pick up traffic or persons coming in from the side. They are seen long before they "pop" into the field of view. There are no surprises, no sudden appearances of previously unseen objects. Things seen far ahead by persons with normal vision come into view for the bioptic user during scanning movements. The normally sighted and the bioptic user both see moving targets closer than one block ahead with peripheral vision. There **is** no jack-in-the-box effect!

A 22-Percent Loss of Field

Years ago, Gerald Fonda, M.D., published an article asserting that the scope causes a 22-percent loss of field vision when it is **not in use.** This is the most outrageous objection of all!

Dr. Fonda speaks from a position of authority as an ophthalmologist. Even when the scope is not in use, it sits there with its silhouette blocking off 22 percent of a driver's vision. This sounds terrible, and it is true. But once again, it is scare tactics. The 22-percent loss of field is five to ten degrees **above the horizon.** It blocks one's view of the sky. The user of the bioptic is only in danger of hitting a low-flying pigeon.

A Proposal for Licensing Visually Impaired Drivers

I do not maintain that all persons with visual impairment should drive. Most low-vision specialists estimate that 6 to 10 percent of the partially sighted stand a chance of getting a license. If only those under age fifty are considered, as stated earlier, I think the percentage is much higher. Using the bioptic does not make someone an unsafe driver.

My work required driving fifty thousand miles a year. I dealt exclusively with the partially sighted. When clients learned I could drive, they often lost interest in other aids. They wanted to drive! This desire is understandable, and I deeply empathized with those who lacked the vision or other abilities to make driving possible.

It was necessary for me to say to some, "No, you shouldn't try to obtain a license." Losing one's independent mobility is a terrible thing, but licensing those who cannot measure up in areas other than vision would be a serious mistake. There are others, however, who can drive with the bioptic. Telescopic glasses are a wonderful driving aid whose "inherent optical deficiencies" are mostly fantasy constructs far removed from the test of reality.

Earlier I briefly discussed the restrictions that states place on drivers using the bioptic. Typically these drivers are restricted to daytime driving, to speeds of forty-five mph or less, and from highway driving. I have pointed out how these restrictions don't make sense. Let me outline how I believe the visually impaired should be tested and licensed.

In some states, low-vision drivers are forced to take the more stringent test given to drivers who lost their licenses for cause. Needless to say, this is unfair.

The low-vision driver will drive where and when he feels confident to drive. This matter of confidence is more important than most people realize. My suggestion is to let the low-vision driver specify where he wants to drive. Then test him in that area. Suppose he wants to drive in his neighborhood and go to the grocery store and to church. Test him over these routes, and issue a license stipulating where he is licensed to drive. Later, or at the same time, if he wants to drive on highways and freeways, or downtown or wherever, retest him and license him accordingly. This kind of testing program makes sense. Having a group of officials, without proper knowledge of either low-vision driving in general or the individual low-vision driver, sitting in a room imposing arbitrary restrictions doesn't make sense.

Officials will claim that they don't have the manpower to do this type of testing, but I happen to know that it is being done already. All over the country, officials give driving tests to persons who cannot pass the vision test. People who are 20/200 (without telescopic glasses) are tested over the roads they want to drive and are issued restricted licenses to do so.

In California, the word is out. A patrolman who knows nothing about vision loss gives the driving test. He sits there, looking like a condemned person about to meet his death, because he thinks he is riding with a blind person. The applicant has on a pair of funny-looking glasses that are supposed to make him safe. If the applicant uses the glasses properly — that is, only when they are needed — he or she risks failing the test, because the patrolman giving the test assumes the driver didn't use the scope often enough. Like I said, the word is out to the visually impaired community: "Keep using the scope even if you don't need it." Unfortunately, this is a wrong — and potentially dangerous — message for so-called public-safety officials to be sending. The roads would be safer if these same officials instead became educated about the realities of driving with subnormal vision, and then updated the regulations to provide for a reasonable method of licensing the visually impaired to drive.

Epilogue

I began my professional life as a Baptist minister — an evangelist of the Gospel (which comes from the Greek word for "good news"). When Stargardt's disease began destroying my vision, I was lucky enough to find help from a good low-vision specialist. I ultimately took a new direction. I became an evangelist of low-vision aids, spreading the good news that the visually impaired can overcome the devastating consequences of vision loss.

The last thirty years have been very rewarding — thousands have heard this gospel and gone on to live productive lives despite vision loss. This is my wish for you. If you read and incorporate into your life the skills and coping techniques discussed in this book, you can vastly improve your situation. Believe it. Do it!

For years I have served as a consultant for persons who have lost some or most of their vision. I extend this service to any person who reads this book. As long as I am alive, I will answer personal questions you may have about your situation.

Bill G. Chapman
Lubbock, Texas
E-mail: chapman@windmill.net

An Eye Test Chart

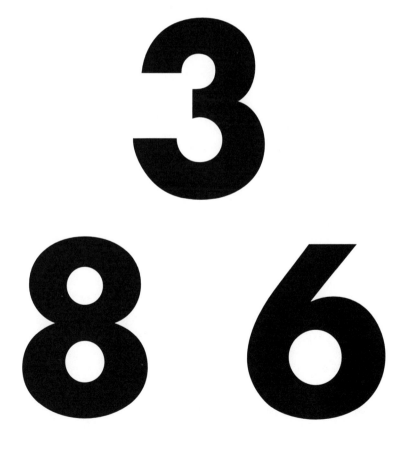

Sources of Help

American Academy of Ophthalmology
655 Beech Street
PO Box 7424
San Francisco CA 94120-7424
(415) 561-8500

Maintains a nationwide list of ophthalmologists who provide low-vision services.

American Academy of Optometry
4330 E. West Hwy #1117
Bethesda MD 20814
(301) 718-6500

Maintains a nationwide list of optometrists who provide low-vision services.

American Foundation for the Blind
11 Penn Plaza, Suite 300
New York NY 10001
(800) 232-5463
New York residents: (212) 502-7657

Maintains a list of low-vision specialists and other services for the visually impaired.

American Optometric Association

243 North Lindbergh Blvd.

St. Louis MO 63141

(314) 991-4100

Maintains a nationwide list of optometrists who specialize in low vision.

American Printing House for the Blind

1839 Frankfort Ave.

Louisville KY 40206

(800) 223-1839

Provides wide-line paper for the visually impaired as well as other products and services. Write or call for a catalog.

Association for Macular Diseases, Inc.

210 East 64th Street

New York NY 10021

(212) 605-3719

A support group for people with macular disease. Publishes a newsletter keeping members informed of research. Dues are $20 per year.

Beecher Research Co.

906 Morse Ave.

Schaumburg IL 60193

(800) 934-8765

Provides binoculars in head-borne frames for watching TV and other distance-viewing tasks.

Bossert Specialties

PO Box 15441

Phoenix AZ 85060

(602) 956-6637

Supplies low-vision aids of many types. Write or call for a catalog. Query them by phone about the price of any aid mentioned in this book. No prescription required.

Corning Medical Optic
Corning Glass Works
PO Box 1511
Elmira NY 14902
(800) 742-5273

A source for doctors to order amber lenses for indoor or outdoor use.

Designs for Vision, Inc.
760 Koehoer Ave.
Ronkonkoma NY 11779
(800) 345-4009

A source for doctors to order telescopic and magnifying spectacles in all powers. They will provide names of doctors who fit their aids.

Enhanced Vision Systems
(800) 440-9476
Website: www.enhancedvision.com

Manufacturer of Jordy glasses.

Expect to Win Enterprises
PO Box 43142
Austin TX 78745-0142
(512) 314-5794

Distributes the book Challenged to Win, by Nancy K. Shugart. Offers inspirational presentations for children and adults who face the challenge of disability.

Humanware
6245 King Rd.

Loomis CA 95650

(800) 722-3393

Provides high-quality video visual aids and other low-vision products.

Independent Living Aids
27 East Mall

Plainview NY 11803-4404

(800) 537-2118

One of the best suppliers of nonprescription low-vision aids. Call or write for a catalog.

LS&S Group, Inc.
PO Box 673

Northbrook IL 60065

(800) 468-4789

A supplier of nonprescription low-vision aids. Write or phone for a catalog.

Macular Degeneration International
Contact person: Tom Perski

6700 N. Oracle Rd., Suite 121

Tucson AZ 85704

(800) 393-7634

A support group for persons with macular degeneration. Dues are $25 a year. One division is devoted to Stargardt's disease, and a second to age-related macular degeneration and other macular problems. Provides many services.

Maxi Aids
PO Box 3209
Farmingdale NY 11735
(800) 522-6249

Supplies nonprescription low-vision aids of all types. Call or write for a catalog.

New York Lighthouse for the Blind
Optical Aids Service
3602 Northern Boulevard
Long Island City NY 11101
(800) 453-4923

Supplies low-vision aids of all types from many manufacturers. Doctor's prescription required for all magnifiers and other aids. Best prices anywhere. They also offer consumer products (nonoptical aids) for the visually impaired that do not require a prescription. Write or call for a catalog.

New York Times Large Print Weekly
(800) 631-2580

Selections from the New York Times newspaper published weekly in large print and mailed to subscribers.

Optelec
PO Box 729
Westford MA 01886
(800) 828-1056

Supplies high-quality video visual aids.

Reader's Digest Large Type Edition
PO Box 241
Mt. Morris IL 61054-9982
(815) 734-6963

Reader's Digest magazine in large print.

Recordings for the Blind
20 Roszel Road
Princeton NJ 08540
(609) 452-0606
Toll-free for registered users only: (800) 221-4792

Provides recorded educational books for students from fourth grade through college and for graduates who want to stay current in their fields.

Recreational Innovation, Inc.
PO Box 159
South Lyon MI 48178
(800) 521-9746

Manufacturer of NOIR sunglasses. Supplies replacements for broken or badly scratched NOIR sunglasses. (Always first try to return damaged glasses to the retailer. Damaged glasses must be returned to be replaced.)

RP Foundation Fighting Blindness, Inc.
Executive Plaza 1, Suite 800
11350 McCormick Rd.
Hunt Valley MD 21031-1014
(800) 683-5555

A support group for persons with RP and related diseases. Offers a newsletter, the names of doctors who provide genetic counseling, and sources of help in dealing with the disease. No dues; a contribution gets you on the mailing list. Also interested in macular degeneration; one of the best sources of information about research in macular degeneration.

Seeing Technology
7070 Brooklyn Blvd.
Brooklyn Center MN 55429
(800) 462-3738

Supplies high-quality video visual aids.

Tech Optics
7893 Enterprise Dr.
Mentor OH 44060
(800) 345-8655

Provides glass microscopes (magnifying spectacles) of exceptional quality in powers up to +100 D. Supplies to doctors only.

Telesensory
520 Almanor Ave.
Sunnydale CA 94086-3533
(800) 804-8004

Supplies electronic aids for the totally blind and the partially sighted.

TIME Magazine Large print Edition
(800) 552-3773 to order a subscription.

Wilmer Low Vision Clinic
Wilmer Eye Institute
550 North Broadway
Baltimore MD 21205
(410) 955-0580

Contact them for information about dealers of the LVES system.

APPENDIX C

Instructions for Building a Plate Light

The light is simply a dry-cell battery attached to a bulb of proper type positioned with copper tubing. It is portable, and can be used in low-light restaurants to illuminate the diner's plate (hence the name "plate light") or menu. Radio Shack part numbers are used to assist in locating needed supplies.

Needed tools include: a drill with a quarter-inch bit, two small screws, lightweight insulated wire, and either electrical or friction tape.

The base is a 6-volt dry cell battery, no. 23-016. The bulb is a no. 40, 6-volt bulb, no. 2721128. The bulb socket is an E-10, miniature threaded base, no.272357. The stand supporting the bulb is $1/4$-inch copper tubing 12 to 15 inches long. Cut a wooden block measuring $1^1/2$ inches square from a 1x2 for the base supporting the socket.

Drill a $1/4$-inch hole in the center of the $1^1/2$-inch-square wooden block. Run two insulated wires through the copper tubing; bend the tubing to shape. Connect the wires to the socket. Pull the slack out of the wires. Screw the E-10 threaded base to the wood. Slip the wooden block over the copper tubing. If the friction fit is not tight enough, coat both surfaces with epoxy glue and let it dry. Stand the copper tubing beside the battery and wrap tape around both to secure the tubing in place. Bring one wire up to connect to the battery post. Leave the other loose until the light is needed. To turn the light on, attach the other wire.

This describes the simplest approach. The light could be made fancier by constructing a wooden case for the battery and wiring in a switch. Make a shade for the bulb with cardboard tacked or glued to the wooden block. Line the inside of the cardboard with aluminum foil to make a reflector.

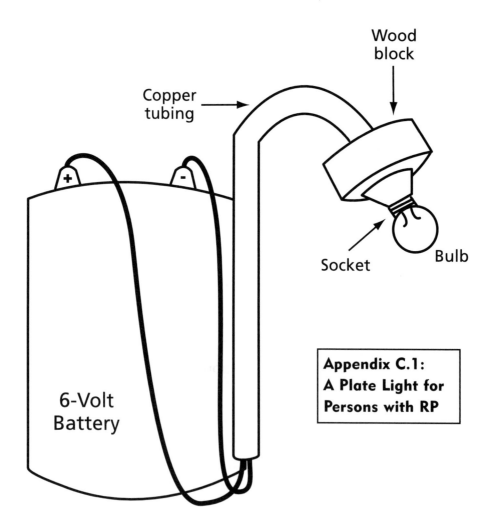

Wood block

Copper tubing

Socket

Bulb

6-Volt Battery

**Appendix C.1:
A Plate Light for
Persons with RP**

Endnotes

1.   This material originally appeared in the author's book <u>Coping with Macular Degeneration</u>, self-published in 1988 by Vision Loss Technology. Permission was granted in November 1990 to the Institute for the Visually Impaired, Department of Graduate Studies in Visual Impairment, Pennsylvania College of Optometry, Philadelphia, to reproduce this chapter in a notebook prepared for their patients.

2.   The source for most of the data in this chapter was material supplied by the RP Foundation Fighting Blindness, Inc.

3.   Material in this chapter was first published in the author's book <u>Coping with Macular Degeneration</u>. Permission was granted in September 1989 to Montana Low Vision Services, Inc., in Helena, to reproduce the material for their clients.

4.   This chapter was first published in the <u>Journal of Rehabilitative Optometry</u>, Fall 1984. The text reproduced here incorporates minor revisions and additions.

5.   This chapter was first published in the <u>Journal of Rehabilitative Optometry</u>, Winter 1984. The text reproduced here incorporates minor revisions and additions.

Bibliography

Factual material in this book grew out of my experience spanning thirty years, including twenty-three years working with people with vision loss. I am indebted to many optometrists, ophthalmologists, and especially low-vision specialists who, formally or informally, taught me the subject.

Two doctors who deserve special recognition are Don Swick, O.D., of El Paso, Texas, who died in January 1999; and Lin Moore, O.D. (retired), of Muskogee, Oklahoma. I and thousands of others owe a debt of gratitude to these two low-vision specialists. The services they performed over the decades for persons with low vision are a living memorial to their skill, knowledge, and commitment to the visually impaired. They were also great teachers who patiently let me pick their brains for information I needed for myself and my clients. Low-vision work came into its own as a specialty during the early 1980s. By that time, these two pioneers were nearing retirement. They had done this work for most of their professional careers.

I consulted several books and other sources to ensure that my knowledge of the diseases discussed in Chapters 8 through 12 was correct and current.

Eden, John. The Physician's Guide to Cataracts, Glaucoma, and Other Eye Problems. Yonkers, NY: Consumer's Reports Books, 1992.

Kelman, Charles D. Cataracts: What You Must Know About Them. Boston, MA: G. K. Hall, 1983.

Leyonecker, W. <u>All About Glaucoma: Questions and Answers for People with Glaucoma</u>. Translated from the German by Alan Pitts. London and Boston, MA: Faber and Faber, 1981.

<u>Living with Low Vision</u>. Lexington, MA: Resources for Rehabilitation, 1993.

Lodewick, Peter A. <u>The Diabetic Man</u>. Los Angeles: Lowell House; Chicago, IL: Contemporary Books, 1991.

Sardegna, Jill and T. Otis Paul. <u>The Encyclopedia of Blindness and Vision Impairment</u>. New York: Facts on File, c. 1991.

Shulman, Julius. <u>Cataracts: The Complete Guide from Diagnosis to Recovery for Patients and Families</u>. New York: Simon and Schuster, 1984.

Subad-Sharpe, Genell J. <u>Living with Diabetes</u>. Garden City, NY: Doubleday, 1985.

Additional Resources

Macular Degeneration International provided some of the information about Stargardt's disease presented in Chapter 11. They also provided the statistical information about macular degeneration presented in Chapter 11.

RP Foundation Fighting Blindness, Inc. provided most of the material presented in Chapter 12.

Index

written by a coalition of the foremost experts

COMPUTER AND WEB RESOURCES FOR PEOPLE WITH DISABILITIES: A Guide to Exploring Today's Assistive Technology   Revised 3rd Edition

by the Alliance for Technology Access

This edition is updated with information about the World Wide Web and its role in expanding human ability and potential.

Part One describes conventional and assistive technologies, and gives strategies for accessing the Internet for education, employment and recreation. It explains how to determine your needs and obtain funding. Personal stories provide examples of how people with different abilities use assistive technology.

Part Two is the "Technology Toolbox," featuring easy-to-use charts organized by key access concerns and referenced to descriptions of software, hardware and communication aids. These include screen enhancers, speech synthesizers, programmable keyboards, switches and much more. Providing the highest level of usability, this Toolbox is organized according to the desired function, not by disability (e.g., by the need to see very large characters on the screen instead of by visual disability or by learning disability).

Part Three tells the reader exactly where to turn for support, information and specific products. It provides a comprehensive list of specialty organizations, funding sources, conferences, government programs, publications, telecommunications resources and technology vendors.

The **Alliance for Technology Access** is a network of resource centers dedicated to providing information and support services for children and adults with disabilities and increasing their use of standard and assistive technologies. Centers can be found nationwide and through the Alliance website at **www.ATAccess.org**

Paperback $20.95 ... Spiral bound $27.95 ... 384 pages ... 8 charts 40 b/w photos ... 7¼ x 9¼

Call if you need help using our order form

ORDER FORM

10% DISCOUNT on orders of $50 or more —
20% DISCOUNT on orders of $150 or more —
30% DISCOUNT on orders of $500 or more —
On cost of books for fully prepaid orders

NAME

ADDRESS

CITY/STATE   ZIP/POSTCODE

PHONE   COUNTRY (outside of U.S.)

TITLE	QTY	PRICE	TOTAL
***Coping with Vision Loss (paperback)*		@ $16.95	

Prices subject to change without notice

Please list other titles below:

		@ $	
		@ $	
		@ $	
		@ $	
		@ $	
		@ $	
		@ $	
		@ $	

Check here to receive our book catalog   ❑   free

Shipping Costs

First book: $3.00 by bookpost, $4.50 by UPS, Priority Mail, or to ship outside the U.S.
Each additional book: $1.00
For rush orders and bulk shipments call us at (800) 266-5592

TOTAL	_____
Less discount @____%	(_____)
TOTAL COST OF BOOKS	_____
CA residents add 7½% sales tax	_____
Shipping & handling	_____
TOTAL ENCLOSED	_____

Please pay in U.S. funds only

❑ Check ❑ Money Order ❑ Visa ❑ Mastercard ❑ Discover

Card #_____ Exp. date_____

Signature_____

Complete and mail to:

Hunter House Inc., Publishers

PO Box 2914, Alameda CA 94501-0914
Website: www.hunterhouse.com
Orders: (800) 266-5592 or email: ordering@hunterhouse.com
Phone (510) 865-5282 Fax (510) 865-4295

CVL- 3/2001